THE DIET CODE

4 STEPS TO PERMANENT WEIGHT LOSS

THE DIET CODE

4 STEPS TO PERMANENT WEIGHT LOSS

DR. MICHAEL IMANI

SPECIAL FIELD ORDER PRESS

Printed in America

Dr. Michael Imani
P.O. Box 56147
Atlanta, Georgia 30343

www.michaelimani.com

TO MY WIFE, DEBBIE...

Thank you for the time you have shared with me, you have never failed to be a beacon of strength and commitment, it is for these reasons and countless others that I dedicate this book to you.

I wish you the very best. I would say 'of luck' - but it really isn't - it's raw persistence and a drive towards your goal and the knowledge that nothing less will do. Look after yourself and keep in touch.

Thomas Chalmers

NOTICE TO READERS

All persistent symptoms, regardless of nature, may have an underlying cause that needs and should not be treated without professional evaluation. It is therefore imperative that if you intend to use this self-help book, only do so in conjunction with duly prescribed advice and consultation. In any event, pay particular attention to the precautions and warnings especially in the section on Autogenics. These precautions advise against anyone experiencing or having experienced the following conditions from using the stress management portion of this book.

THERE ARE SEVERAL PRECAUTIONS TO CONSIDER PRIOR TO LEARNING AUTOGENICS .

ALTHOUGH (AT) AUTOGENICS IS A RATHER SIMPLE TECHNIQUE, IT IS A VERY POWERFUL ONE. CONSEQUENTLY, IT MAY NOT BE SUITABLE FOR EVERYONE. YOU SHOULD ALWAYS LEARN THE METHOD FROM A QUALIFIED INSTRUCTOR WHENEVER POSSIBLE. AUTOGENICS SHOULD NOT BE UNDERTAKEN UNDER "ANY" OF THE FOLLOWING CIRCUMSTANCES:

1. During or immediately following a heart attack (acute myocardial infraction),

2. If you are a diabetic undergoing insulin treatment, because insulin consumption and utilization may swing wildly during AT (which results in the need for constant monitoring of both blood and urine therefore it is ill-advised for the majority of diabetics),

3. If you suffer glaucoma,

4. If you suffer from psychotic conditions such as schizophrenia or severe depression associated with hallucinations or feelings of unreality,

5. If you have had electric shock treatment,

6. If you are an active alcoholic or drug abuser,

7. If you suffer from epilepsy, or

8. If you have ever had a prolonged episode of unconsciousness,

If you do not fall into any of these categories, then there is no reason why you should not be able to begin Autogenics.

ACKNOWLEDGMENTS

I want to first acknowledge the immeasurable contributions of the late Drs Johannes W. Schultz and Wolfgang Luthe, without whom autogenics would likely have never been conceptualized. I would also like to thank one of the great figures in the history of AT, the late famed British psychotherapists, Vera Diamond. She was a personal mentor and heroine.

I would like to also thank Laura Brooks, Dr. Jelani Madaraka, Amsa Shepsu, Gary Clement, Dr. Alex Docker, Julie Rainbow and countless others who inspired me along this journey. A special note of thanks to one of the greatest coaches on the planet and a personal friend of mine, Thomas Chalmers.

Finally, I would like to thank each of my clients over the years for being great teachers in their own unique ways.

TABLE OF CONTENTS

Chapters

Introduction

David ate what he wanted, when he wanted. I was like David. He said, "I ate at all the wrong times and the wrong foods at all the wrong times." David ended up tipping the scale at 525 pounds. He stated, "I couldn't take 10 steps without stopping to take deep breaths," "Stairs were out of the question. It just made it difficult to do everything." This led David to seek a *different choice*. This was <u>how</u> he would do it.

Instead of chasing the latest fad diet, he decided to take the longer, steadier path to better health. David **lost 305 pounds in one year and 17 days.** He says, "....I did it the right way," "I ate a lot of the right foods and I exercised every day." The old meals of a large pizza, a 12-inch sub and a 2-liter soda were in the past.

He also changed how he used his spare time. He would use weights while watching television. David Caruso lost 305 pounds and 36 inches off his waist in one year and 17 days.

He *credits a mindset change in how he wanted his life to be.* He said, "I always tried to convince myself (that) it's not a diet, it's a lifestyle, (and) that you're going to have to live the rest of your life (sticking to it). That's what I did." This book and this approach to permanent weight loss is dedicated to my clients and those heros like David.

INTRODUCTION

The Current Reality

At the present time more people on this planet struggle with being overweight and obese than at any other time in history. Experts project that seven in ten American men will be overweight at some point in their adult lives. For women, that number is projected to be nine in ten.

We all have heard the grim statistics of how many people fail to succeed on diets each year. The commercial weight loss industry has a 95% failure rate. Yet the industry will earn almost $50,000,000,000.00 (50 billion) this year alone. Sadly, dieters have better odds at Las Vegas or Atlantic City - 95 or every 100 people lose by failing to permanently lose.

So, why do so many people fall into this trap repeatedly? Or, perhaps a better question is, "Why do people find it so difficult to lose weight when it does not have to be difficult?" There are a range of answers to this question. For many, they are doing all the right things in one area, say exercise, but they are eating too many calories to support weight loss. Or, they might be doing some things great, but they will rarely see the results they desire without doing all things consistently. For many, they don't even know that a code exists. Most don't even know there is a code to permanent weight loss.

All of this comes down to the fact that people who struggle with weight simply do not know the code. Your success depends on four factors. Diet, Exercise, Accountability, and Stress management.

This code is built on these four success factors and this book will tell you *exactly* what to do in each of these four areas to produce permanent results.

I have discovered that losing weight does not have to be a struggle. It does not have to be a burden or some scarlet letter. I have discovered a code. This code I refer to unlocks this secret to permanent weight loss. It is simple. I have boiled it down to a simple ten-digit number. That is correct. If you can remember a telephone number, then you can lose as much weight as you like, and keep it off permanently. This is the guarantee of the Diet Code.

A SIMPLE TEN-DIGIT PHONE NUMBER?

After years of research and several years of working with clients, I have translated these facts into a simple ten-digit telephone number, a diet code.

Each ten-digit code is made up of specific daily habits that you do at very specific times and in very specific amounts. The research and clinical experience suggests that you must do very specific things on a consistent basis in order to lose weight *permanently*. Once you accept this idea and understand how each digit of the number supports the overall code, then you will be able to simply follow the daily steps by following the telephone number.

Each of these specific behavioral factors have been combined to create these codes. All you then have to do is to follow what your code lays out and three things will happen: 1) You will stop gaining weight, 2) You will begin to lose weight, and 3) You will be able to permanently live within your healthy weight range.

THE DIET CODE PHILOSOPHY

This book is more a how-to manual than a nutritional guide, although it does contain some aspects that speak to nutrition. Most of the book is about your life and reconciling gaps in your life. In other words, I believe that you must put your weight into the larger context of your life in order to find a permanent solution. David knew this, I know this, and I believe you know this. I further believe that any approach to weight loss, especially permanent weight loss, must be three (3) things: *safe, simple, and sustainable.*

Safety.

We all can remember the shock of people actually dying in the "phen fen" days. Part of my client roster is people who are "morbidly or clinically obese." Many of these clients have been advised to consider weight-loss surgery, which is not without serious risk. A 2005 study by researchers at the University of Washington found that 1 in 50 people die within one month of having gastric bypass surgery, and that figure jumps nearly five-fold if the surgeon is inexperienced. One of my clients was advised within two minutes of meeting a doctor for the first time, that they should consider surgery. The doctor had never seen her before nor was he familiar with her medical history, but he had a referral ready within minutes. This program is safe and natural - no pills, shakes, powders, and no magic solutions or games.

Simplicity.

Let's be honest here. We all are seeking the most for the least. Not unlike shopping for a new home or a new car. As I have said, I know people who kill themselves in the gym but then eat all the wrong things in the wrong amounts and wonder why they don't enjoy the desired results. This program operates off the basic idea that if you can get the desired results by exercising 18 minutes per day, then you should exercise 18 minutes. If it is 68 minutes for you, it is 68 minutes. I have determined through real-life experience with clients and research that this program produces permanent results that are safe, sustainable, and simple. If you want a program that is simple and fits into your life then, the Diet Code is for you.

Sustainability.

I suspect you also are seeking solutions that are sustainable. Perhaps you, like me for years, would yo-yo up and down, gaining, losing, and regaining the same pounds. This program was built so that you can begin it early in life and could be still living the code in your 90's. I am a baby boomer and my generation is looking for sustainable solutions to this question. I stopped running years ago, not because I could not but because I recognized that running would not be sustainable for *me* over time. As a result, I began to seek out exercises that would not impact my joints such as swimming, rowing, and walking.

I am in the business of providing my clients *permanent,* sustainable solutions. Many of them start at weights over 350 pounds, and the only thing they can do is water aerobics as their knees will not support even walking for 5 minutes much less sixty. However, they are surprised at how quickly they are regularly walking for an hour. Just take the first step, it will be the most difficult one but it will be a *sustainable* one. The commercial diet industry is a GREAT business to be in at this time in history if you are into that type of thing. However, I believe that your dreams are too important to risk to chance, they are too important to leave to a game that is stacked against you, but there is a permanent solution, the Diet Code.

6 STEPS TO USING THE DIET CODE

Step 1.

First determine **your <u>present</u> weight and starting calorie level**. I underscore your <u>present</u> weight because as you lose weight, and move from stage 1 to 2 for example, your code will then change from 1600 to 1400 if you are a female and from 1800 to 1600 if you are a male. Determine your present weight with a digital scale.

weight	female	male	stage
301 and over	1600 calories	1800 calories	1
251 to 300	1400 calories	1600 calories	2
250 and less	1200 calories	1400 calories	3

Step 2.

Then - based on your starting calorie level and gender, **identify your *beginning* code**.

code	female	male
1800	n/a	876-554-6083
1600	865-553-6083	865-553-6083
1400	854-443-6083	854-443-6083
1200	843-343-6083	n/a

Step 3.

Next, **learn what each digit represents.** For example, regardless of what your code is, digit #4 will always represent the number of portions of fresh organic fruits you will eat daily. Each digit represents a specific daily behavior or action, which will be measured when you record your daily code. In the example below, I use the 1800 code. If you fully complete each daily code as designed, you will begin to lose weight and you will continue to lose weight consistently until you reach your goal.

each digit in all codes represents a specific activity	categories	e.g. 1800 code: [876-554-6083] (daily portions)
digit #1	pure water	8
digit #2	whole grains	7
digit #3	protein/dairy	6
digit #4*	fresh organic fruits	5 *(or more)
digit #5*	organic vegetables	5 *(or more)
digit #6	healthy fats	4
digits #7&8	aerobic exercise	60 minutes
digit #9	strength training	8 minutes
digit #10	stress management	3 sessions
876-554-6083		876-554-6083

Step 4.

Set up *a two-stage accountability system.*

Stage 1 requires you to "get some skin into the game," by risking something emotionally. This means identifying the person that you would rather die than to let down or fail. This can't be you because you would not be reading this book if you had kept faith with yourself. This could be your spouse, your child, your children, your Mother, your Father, your lover, your colleagues,or your coach. I don't care, just look them in the eye and make a promise. Then *keep the promise.*

I, _____, promise you,

_____, that I will reach the goal I have set for myself and I know I am confidently moving toward it each day. I need your support and your help. I will share my results by **weighing every Monday and Friday** until I celebrate my one year anniversary of reaching my goal and maintaining my weight within my healthy weight range.

Signature

_____

Date _____

Look at this promise and carry it with you everyday until you reach your goal weight plus one year. Additionally, you should photocopy this and provide your coach with a copy.

Stage 2 requires you to establish daily and weekly benchmarks. As students are taught in Business school, "If you can measure it, you can change it." Each day you must record your actual code for the day and you will conduct a weekly (monday - sunday) assessment of the results. This is an actual week for me where you can see how I have both documented the code and how I did for the week in terms of actual targets and goals for each digit of the Diet Code.

	8	7	6	5	5	4	60	8	3	wt.
mon	8	6	6	4	4	4	60	8	3	188
tue	8	6	5	5	4	3	60	8	3	
wed	11	7	5	4	5	4	60	8	2	
thur	10	6	6	5	6	3	60	8	3	
fri	6	8	6	5	4	5	60	0	2	187
sat	8	6	2	7	4	3	60	8	4	
sun	7	5	7	5	8	5	60	0	1	
%	58/56	44/49	37/42	35/35	35/35	27/28	360/360	40/56	18/21	
	104	90%	88%	100	100	96%	100	71%	86%	

It is critically important for you to sit down every week to review the past week, focus on the one area that you will make improve on the upcoming week (for me it would have been in the 9th digit, strength training, *71%), and offer gratitude for a successful week even before it arrives. You can do this by visualizing or imagining and experiencing the positive emotion of a great week - even before it gets here.

digit #1 - water	104%
digit #2 - whole grains	90%
digit #3 - protein/dairy	88%
digit #4 - fruits	100%
digit #5 - vegetables	100%
digit #6 - healthy fats	96%
digits 7&8 - aerobic exercise	100%
digit #9 - strength training	*71%
digit #10- stress management	86%

Plan for and ensure that you have weekly time with your coach to discuss how you are to continue moving forward.

Step 5.

Identify your beginning calorie code tracking sheet on one of the following four pages. Each sheet will track your results for a two-week period. Then simply follow and record the code each day noting your weight on each Monday and Friday mornings. Be sure to plan the upcoming week on each Sunday with your coach after you complete your efficiency percentages for each category. Photocopy each of these pages as you lose weight and move through stages.

Step 6.

Begin week one of AT practice at the start of your third week.

1800 CALORIE DIET CODE

	8	7	6	5+	5+	4	60	8	3	wt.
mon	w	w	p	f	v	f	w	s	a	?
tue	a	h	r	r	e	a	a	t	u	
wed	t	o	o	u	g	t	l	r	t	
thur	e	l	t	i	e	s	k	e	o	
fri	r	e	e	t	t		i	n	g	?
sat			i	s	a		n	g	e	
sun		g	n		b		g	t	n	
%		r	s		l			h	i	
mon		a	&		e				c	?
tue		i	d		s			t	s	
wed		n	a					r		
thur		s	i					a		
fri			r					i		?
sat			y					n		
sun										
%										

copy and use this sheet to track your results

1600 CALORIE DIET CODE

	8	6	5	5+	5+	3	60	8	3	wt.
mon	w	w	p	f	v	f	w	s	a	?
tue	a	h	r	r	e	a	a	t	u	
wed	t	o	o	u	g	t	l	r	t	
thur	e	l	t	i	e	s	k	e	o	
fri	r	e	e	t	t		i	n	g	?
sat			i	s	a		n	g	e	
sun		g	n		b		g	t	n	
%		r	s		l			h	i	
mon		a	&		e				c	?
tue		i	d		s			t	s	
wed		n	a					r		
thur		s	i					a		
fri			r					i		?
sat			y					n		
sun										
%										

copy and use this sheet to track your results

1400 CALORIE DIET CODE

	8	5	4	4+	4+	3	60	8	3	wt.
mon	w	w	p	f	v	f	w	s	a	?
tue	a	h	r	r	e	a	a	t	u	
wed	t	o	o	u	g	t	l	r	t	
thur	e	l	t	i	e	s	k	e	o	
fri	r	e	e	t	t		i	n	g	?
sat			i	s	a		n	g	e	
sun		g	n		b		g	t	n	
%		r	s		l			h	i	
mon		a	&		e				c	?
tue		i	d		s			t	s	
wed		n	a					r		
thur		s	i					a		
fri			r					i		?
sat			y					n		
sun										
%										

copy and use this sheet to track your results

1200 CALORIE DIET CODE

	8	4	3	3+	4+	3	60	8	3	wt.
mon	w	w	p	f	v	f	w	s	a	?
tue	a	h	r	r	e	a	a	t	u	
wed	t	o	o	u	g	t	l	r	t	
thur	e	l	t	i	e	s	k	e	o	
fri	r	e	e	t	t		i	n	g	?
sat			i	s	a		n	g	e	
sun		g	n		b		g	t	n	
%		r	s		l			h	i	
mon		a	&		e				c	?
tue		i	d		s			t	s	
wed		n	a					r		
thur		s	i					a		
fri			r					i		?
sat			y					n		
sun										
%										

copy and use this sheet to track results

IMPORTANT POINTS BEFORE YOU START

Weighing. You will weigh on Monday and Friday mornings [on a digital scale] _before_ either drinking or eating _anything_, in the _nude_, and _after_ urinating and having a morning bowel movement(s). I stress a digital reading because of the accuracy of the measurement. In this program or any responsible one, your goal should be approximately two (2) pounds of body fat per week. However, as David's example showed us, it is possible to safely lose more.

Eating. You will note that I do suggest, in the strongest terms, foods you should avoid and those that you should build your diet around. These "better" choices are identified _by type and **specific portion sizes according to each digit in later chapters.**_ You already know which foods contribute to the problem. As long as you follow the plan that is presented here, you will succeed. Remember, "Skin in the game." This program is about you making better choices in every area of your life, beginning with your weight. _You MUST learn portions to be successful._ **_You will need a small food scale to measure your meats, a one cup, a one-half cup, and a one-third cup container until you know exactly what 3 ounces of meat is or what 1/2 cup of beans really looks like._** _Refer to each chapter or digit until you know and recognize what a portion really is._

. **you must eat every 2.5 to 3 hours with the goal of eating 5 to 6 meals each day.** _If you do not, you body will fight to hold onto fat because it believes that you are starving. Therefore, you can workout everyday, but you will not lose weight and keep it off ever. You must eat every couple of hours to keep your metabolism burning fat. Period._

. you **must eat breakfast within 30 minutes of your morning 8 minute workout.** Also, your last meal must be eaten no later than 10 p.m. (preferably by 8 p.m.).

digit 1

Water

The
1st digit in the Diet Code
always represents the number of **8**
ounce glasses of *water* to be consumed
daily. Water contains 0 calories. Each day
you will minimally consume 8 glasses of water regardless of what code or stage you find
yourself ... For each 25 pounds you are
overweight, you should drink an
additional glass.

876-554-6083

The first digit in the Diet Code represents daily water intake. Water may be the most important factor in permanent weight loss. How much water is enough? Well, I will answer that by establishing a baseline that applies to virtually all of us. That is, we should all, regardless of current weight, be drinking a minimum of 64 ounces daily. *However,* if you are overweight, then you need one additional glass for every 25 pounds of excess weight beyond your healthy weight. Cold water is absorbed into the system more quickly than warm water.

Ideally, you should attempt to distribute your water over the course of the entire day, consuming a quart in the morning, a quart during the midday, and a final quart between 5 p.m, and 7 p.m.

The human body is perfectly balanced. When we provide it with the proper water, several things happen:

. fluid retention is alleviated

. your natural thirst returns

. your are less hungry virtually overnight

. more fat is burned as fuel, the liver is then free to metabolize fat, and

. endocrine-gland function improves

On the other hand, if you stop drinking enough water, the delicate balance will be thrown out of balance again, and you are likely to experience fluid retention, unexplained weight gain and loss of thirst. To remedy the situation, you will have to drink enough on a consistent basis to place your body back into balance again.

Water contains zero calories. The health benefits are enormous. The "8" or water portion of the code is placed at the very beginning of the code in an effort to underscore its importance as quite possibly the most critical factor in not only losing weight, but also in keeping it off.

I will briefly make the case here. First, water is a natural appetite suppressant in addition to helping the body metabolize stored body fat. Some studies have found that a decrease water intake will result in an increase in fat storage. Whereas, an increase in water intake actually results in a reduction in stored fat. This is because your kidneys can't function properly without enough water. When this happens, the kidneys do not work to full capacity. As a result, some of their workload is then shifted to the liver.

Well, one of your liver's central jobs is to metabolize stored body fat by converting it into usable energy for your body. However, if the liver has to stop and help the kidneys, it can not operate at full efficiency. As a result, it metabolizes less fat, and more fat remains stored in the body. And, yes, you stop losing weight.

Many people experience fluid retention. Drinking adequate water is the best remedy for fluid retention. What happens when you don't drink enough? Well, the same thing that occurs when you eat only three meals each day. Your body, which can not on its own understand that there is a clean water source about every few feet in any direction, perceives this as a threat to its survival and it begins to hold onto every single drop it can. Since water is stored in the extra-cellular spaces surrounding cells, this often shows up in the form of swollen legs, hands, and feet. All of which means extra pounds. <u>I have seen clients have seven pound "water weight" increases in weight after a bag of salted popcorn at the movie.</u> Many people seek the band aid fix of diuretics by forcing this stored water out (along with essential nutrients). Again, the body perceives a threat and will replace this lost water at the first opportunity. So, you have not solved the problem.

The best way of addressing the problem of your body retaining water is to simply provide it more water. It is only then that it will release what it has stored. If fluid retention is a recurring theme in your life, then you must look at the prime suspect, salt. Because of the finely tuned balance of your body, it will only tolerate sodium in specific concentrations. So, the more salt you eat, the more water your body will retain in order to dilute it. Therefore, the more water you drink, the quicker excess sodium is removed.

It stands to reason that an obese person requires more water than a thin person. Therefore, water being a key factor in the metabolism of fat, overweight people require more water. Water provides additional advantages such as helping to maintain proper muscle tone along with preventing dehydration. It also helps to prevent the problem of sagging skin that is commonly associated with significant weight loss. With proper water intake, shrinking cells are buoyed leaving them full. This results in the appearance of healthy, clear, and strong skin. When you do not get the proper water, the body steals from internal sources. The colon is the primary target. This results in constipation. This is usually and easily corrected by increasing water consumption. Additionally, water helps our body to eliminate waste. During weight loss, the body of course has more waste to eliminate in the form of stored body fat. There is a direct link between water intake and weight loss. Here are the facts:

. Your body can't burn stored fat without proper water intake
. The only way to get rid of excess water is to drink more water.
. Retained water shows up as excess water weight, 7 lbs. in some.
. Drinking water is essential to weight loss.

Daily Water Intake	number of daily 8-ounce glasses of water
1800,1600,1400, & 1200	8 minimal

digit 2

Whole grains

The 2nd digit in the Diet Code always represents the number of portions of *whole grains* to be eaten daily. Each portion equals 70 calories. Each day you will eat either 7, 6, 5, or 4 portions of whole grains depending on what code or stage you are. In this example, we use the 1800 code, which is *7 portions of whole grains daily.

876-554-6083

I have been very deliberate here in my not referring to this category as carbohydrates. I make this distinction because many people who struggle with managing their weight do so in part because they do not fully understand the impact of complex, simple and processed carbohydrates on their blood sugar levels and ultimately on hormonally-driven hunger. I further believe that many people are "hooked" on the rush they get from sugary, processed carbohydrates. This is not an accident.

Consider the example of breads. You should always look for pieces of actual grain in the breads you consume. According to Dr. Andrew Weil, one of the most respected experts in the area of Integrative Medicine in the world, "If you can crush a slice of bread into a marble-size ball, it has a high glycemic load, *whether it looks brown or white.* Low-glycemic-load breads are dense and chewy and full of cracked pieces of grains. Although you may see labels that say 'made with whole grains,' be wary because these products may be made with flour." Weil suggests eating fewer products produced with any kind of flour and eating more whole or cracked grains, such as wild rice, barley, quinoa.

There is broad agreement on the fact that consuming whole grains in their *natural state is generally viewed as something quite different than* eating a white flour alternative or something simply labeled whole wheat or whole grain. It is important for you to know that many products made with "whole grain flour" or "whole grain" are made from pulverized grains not grains still in tact. In their natural state, whole grains are made up of three (3) parts: the bran, the endosperm, and the germ.

What this means is that the bran (the fiber-rich outer layer) and the germ (the nutrient-rich inner part) of the grain have been removed during the milling process The only thing left is the endosperm (the middle part). In the refinement process, many of the B vitamins, iron, vitamin E, selenium, fiber and other disease-fighting components are removed. Even though manufacturers will "enrich" their products with niacin, riboflavin, thiamin, and iron for example, they are not able restore the insoluble fiber and other important nutrients lost during the milling process. More specifically, when grains are milled, the starch is pulverized. This creates a large surface area for the digestive enzymes to work. This results in a very fast conversion to starch and sugar, *which results in an undesirable spike or peak in blood sugar and insulin secretion.* Note the following list of refined grains (Avoid these foods):

. WHITE BREADS
. WHITE RICE
. WHITE FLOUR GOODS
. CRACKERS
. PASTA
. NON-WHOLE GRAIN CEREALS
. PRE-PACKAGED BAKED GOODS

There are very good reasons why your diet should be built around whole grains. Here are a few. Again, whole grains contain the bran, endosperm, and the germ. Since they have not gone through the milling process, they remain good sources of fiber, B vitamins, iron, zinc, magnesium, vitamin E, and selenium. They further contain plant chemicals known as phytochemicals - believed to have many health-promoting effects. Whole grains have been proven to lead to:

. reduced constipation and hemorrhoids
. lower cholesterol levels and decreased the risk of heart disease
. reduced the risk of type 2 diabetes
. increased absorption of nutrients, due to longer digestion

Whole grain portions [70 calories per serving]

. barley, cooked 1/3 cup
. bread, sourdough 1 slice
. bread, whole grain 1 slice
. bulgar, cooked 1/2 cup
. cereal, whole grain 1/2 cup
. whole grain, english muffin 1/2
. oatmeal, cooked 1/2 cup
. baby, red-skinned potatoes 3 small
. rice, brown cooked 1/3 cup
. soup, broth-based 1 cup
. soup, chicken noodle 1 cup
. soup, tomato 1 cup
. soup, vegetable 1 cup

Code	number of daily whole grain portions
1800	7
1600	6
1400	5
1200	4

digit 3

Protein/Dairy

The
3rd digit in the Diet Code
always represents the number of
portions of *protein/dairy* to be eaten
daily. Each portion equals 110 calories.
Every day you will eat either 6, 5, 4 or 3 portions of protein or dairy depending on what
code or stage you are .... For example,
in the 1800 code below, **6** daily
portions are eaten.

87**6**-554-6083

Because of the wide range of approaches to eating, vegan, vegetarian, or carnivore, the code is more concerned with the three main criteria for any diet: safety, sustainability, and simplicity. Today, Americans consume far less red meat than 30 years ago. Although, this figure is still approximately 65 pounds of beef a year.

Beyond recent concerns of E. coli and mad-cow disease, there are health concerns related to pork, beef, veal, and lamb consumption. The poultry industry is presently dealing with the Bird flu virus. There are studies that have linked an increased risk of heart disease to consumption of red meat. On the other hand, there are also studies that clearly have found lower rates of cardiovascular disease amongst people who eat diets lower in red meat consumption.

Preparation is also a factor that should concern you. We know that *grilling, frying, or broiling* animal products in general and red meats in particular can create toxic compounds. These have been found to be linked to increased risk in colorectal, lung, and pancreatic cancers. To reduce these risks, reduce cooking time, select lean cuts, and marinate the cuts.

The high consumption of processed meat options such as hot dogs, luncheon meats, and other choices have been linked to higher risk for developing type 2 diabetes, stroke, pancreatic and colorectal cancer. If giving up meat is not a choice for you, then you may consider these options.

Organic meats labeled 100% organic must meet specific requirements. For instance, beef with this label were only fed organic grass or grain, were not fed any antibiotics or hormones, and were provided access to air, water, and sunshine. This organic label is the only one certified by the USDA.

Lightly pan searing meats with olive or canola oil, or baking provide safer options you may wish to explore.

The following is a list of proteins or dairy representing a wide range of eating approaches. Each serving on the list equals 110 calories.

Protein / dairy portions [110 calories per serving]

. beans 1/2 cup	1/2 cup
. beef, lean 1.5 ounces	1.5 ounces
. chicken, skinless	2.5 ounces
. cheese	

- cheddar, low fat,   2 oz., 1/2 cup
- colby, low fat,   2 oz., shredded 1/2 cup
- cottage, low fat 2/3 cup
- feta 1/4 cup
- mozzarella, part skim, shredded   1/3 cup
- parmesan, grated 4 tsp.
- ricotta, part-skim 1/3 cup
- swiss, low fat 2 oz.

. clams, canned 1/3 cup	
. cod	3 oz.
. crab	3 oz.
. duck, breast	3 oz.
. egg	1 lg.
. egg, substitute	1/2 cup
. egg whites	4
. fish	3 oz.
. garbanzo beans	1/3 cup
. halibut	3 oz.
. ice cream, fat free vanilla	1/2 cup
. lamb, lean no fat	2 oz.
. lentils	1/2 cup

. milk, skim, 1 or 2 %   1 cup
. pheasant   3 oz.
. pork, lean cuts, no fat   2 oz.
. salmon   3 oz.
. scallops   3 oz.
. shrimp   3 oz.
. soybeans, green   1/2 cup
. tofu   1/2 cup
. tempeh   1/3 cup
. tuna, canned, in water   1/2 cup
. turkey   3 oz.
. veal   2 oz.
. veggie bean burger   3 oz.
. venison   3 oz.
. yogurt, fat free, low calorie   1 cup
. yogurt, fat free, frozen   1/2 cup

Code	number of daily protein/ dairy portions
1800	6
1600	5
1400	4
1200	3

digit **4**

Fruits

The
4th digit in the Diet Code
always represents the number of
portions of fresh organic fruits to be eaten
daily based on your code or stage...... In
each code, you will notice that you are always
able to eat as many servings of fruit as you
like each day. In the 1800 code below,
you will note 5 or more servings of
fruit each day.

876-**5**54-6083

Eating *fresh organic* fruits provide tremendous health benefits. We do know that those people who eat more fruits and vegetables (within the context of an overall healthy diet) have a reduced risk of some serious medical conditions and chronic diseases such as stroke and perhaps cardiovascular diseases. Eating a diet rich in fruits and vegetables is part of an overall healthy approach and may protect against certain cancers, such as mouth, stomach, and colon-rectum. Fruits provide you with critical nutrients for the health and maintenance of your body. Finally, fruits will become more tasty and attractive to you as you consume less processed sugar in your diet.

The following is a list of fruits. Each portion is 60 calories per serving.

Fruits

. apple	1 small
. applesauce, unsweetened	1/2 cup
. apricots	4
. banana	1 sm., 1/2 lg.
. berries, mixed	1 cup
. blackberries	1 cup
. blueberries	3/4 cup
. cherries	1 cup/ 1 dz.
. dates	3
. figs, dried	3 small
. figs, fresh	2 small
. grapefruit	1 small/ 1/2 lg.
. grapes	1 cup
. kiwi	1 large

. mixed fruit	3/4 cup
. nectarine	1
. orange	1 medium
. peach	1 large
. pear	1 small
. plums	2
. prunes	3
. raisins	2 tbsp.
. raspberries	1 cup
. strawberries	1 & 1/5 cup
. tangerine	1 large
. watermelon	1 sm. wedge

Code	number of daily fruit portions
1800	5+
1600	5+
1400	4+
1200	3+

digit 5

Vegetables

The
5th digit of the Diet Code always represents the number of portions
of *vegetables* to be eaten daily by you. Each
portion is 25 calories. Each day you will eat
either 4, 5 or more portions of vegetables
depending on what code or stage you
are.....

876-554-6083

Most health experts agree that there is overwhelming evidence that a diet rich in vegetables and fruits help to *prevent most types of cancer.* Vegetables contain compounds that are known antioxidants. These prevent damage to DNA that can trigger cancer.

A recent study found that women with the highest consumption levels of vegetables and fruits had a 43% lower risk of breast cancer recurrence versus women with the lowest intake levels, this according to the Journal of Clinical Oncology.

The list of fresh organic vegetables is seemingly endless: artichokes, asparagus, broccoli, collards, bok choy, kale, sprouts, brussels sprouts, and cabbage just to name a few. I suspect that all of us understand the connection between eating several servings of vegetables and improvements in overall health. One study found that men who ate only five (5) servings *per week* were 10 to 20% less likely to develop prostate cancer. There is a growing body of research evidence that has found lycopene, a pigment found in tomatoes is a powerful antioxidant that may be helpful in defeating cancer. The process of cooking tomatoes is known to release more lycopene than raw ones. Lycopene is also known to reduce inflammation. Vegetables [25 calories per serving]

. artichoke	1/2 bud
. asparagus	1/2 c. / 6 spears
. bean sprouts	1 cup
. beets	1/2 c.
. bell pepper	1 medium
. broccoli	1 cup
. brussels sprouts	4 sprouts
. cabbage, cooked	1 cup
. cabbage, raw	1 cup
. cauliflower	1 cup florets
. celery	4 med. stalks

. cherry, grape tomatoes   8, 1 cup
. cucumber   1 c. sliced, 1 med.
. eggplant, cooked   1 c. pieces
. green beans   3/4 cup
. green onions, scallions   3/4 c., or 8
. kale, cooked   2/3 cup
. lettuce   2 cup, shredded
. mariana sauce   1/4 cup
. mushrooms   1 cup
. okra   1/2c. / 3 pods
. onions   1/2 c. sliced
. peas, green   1/4 cup
. pizza sauce   1/4 cup
. radishes   25 medium
. salsa   1/4 cup
. shallots   3 tbsp.
. spinach, cooked   1/2 cup
. spinach, raw   2 cups
. squash, summer   3/4 cup sliced
. tomatillo   1/2 c. diced
. tomato   1 medium
. water chestnuts   3/4 c.

Code	number of daily vegetable portions
1800	5+
1600	5+
1400	4
1200	4

digit **6**

Healthy Fats

The
6th digit of the Diet Code
always will represent the number of
portions of *healthy fats* consumed daily.
Each portion of fat equals 45 calories. Each
day you will consume either 3 or 4 portions of
fat depending on what code or stage you
find yourself.....

876-554-6083

HEALTHY FATS

In the midst of this current debate on obesity, one of the easy targets has been oils. At about 120 calories per tablespoon, cooking oils, are an easy target.

It has been my experience, which is now supported by a growing body of research, that a diet including adequate amounts of healthy fats actually promotes health. For instance, a diet that includes unsalted organic walnuts, a good quality (extra virgin) olive oil, and fish is considered a healthy approach to fat consumption. But, as we all know, there also exists unhealthy fats.

I make the distinction of "healthy fats" because it will be one of the most important considerations for all of us in today's world of endless food choices. Trans fats, the most dangerous of all, are frequently found in baked goods; deep-fried foods because they are cheap, can be used over and over again, and they dramatically extend the shelf life of the product.

THE DANGER OF TRANS FATS

Trans fats are so dangerous that Los Angeles, New York City, Chicago and a growing list of cities are considering a total ban on them. In fact, in December of 2006, New York City became the first major city in the U.S. to ban trans fats. New York's law requires *all* restaurant food prepared have less that 0.5 grams of synthetic trans fat per serving by July 2008. A total ban of any food in the $900 billion food industry is rare, but in this case, many believe that people's lives are at risk. At present, some cities have strongly encouraged restaurants to reduce trans fats from sources such as partially hydrogenated oils, margarine, and shortening with very little success.

Experts agree that consuming as little as 4 grams daily (a single serving of fries contains 5 grams) significantly increases the risk of heart disease. The problem is that although the FDA requires trans fats be listed on packaging - they do not require this be disclosed by restaurants. At present, it is impossible to determine how much is in that dinner or lunch you just ate.

Experts further agree that trans fats contribute to chronic inflammation, diabetes, cancer, to name a few life threatening conditions. Consider that beyond the known cardiovascular risks trans fats may also increase the risk of fertility problems by more than seventy (70) percent according to a study published in the Journal of Clinical Nutrition.

Trans fats provide no nutritional value. After a seven year delay, fast-food giant McDonald's has begun to use trans-fat-free oil in its french fries in _some_ of its restaurants.

According to the President of the Physicians Committee for Responsible Medicine, Dr. Neal Barnard, M.D., advises ***avoiding pastries and fried foods and choosing vegetarian entrees when dining out.***

HEALTHY FATS

The following represents a list of the healthy fats.

Healthy Fats [45 calories per serving]

. extra virgin olive oil	1 teaspoon
. raw peanut butter	1.5 teaspoons
. canola oil	1 teaspoon
. ground flaxseed	2 teaspoons
. avocado	1/6

. walnuts, organic   4 halves
. almonds, organic   9

Fat is not your enemy in the quest for permanent weight loss. In fact, healthy fats can be essential in not only losing weight but keeping it off also. Perhaps the best oil or fat choice available to any of us is extra virgin olive oil. Making this your number one choice is a healthy and wise choice.

Consider that olive oil is primarily a monounsaturated fat, which lowers LDL, or unhealthy cholesterol while not affecting HDL, healthy or good cholesterol. There is also evidence that olive oil reduces the risk of cancer because of antioxidant-rich compounds. You should only purchase, *extra virgin olive oils, which are gently pressed.* In the Fall of 2004, the FDA agreed to allow manufacturers to claim on food labels that olive oil *may reduce heart disease.* Great for salads and for pan searing meats and vegetables. As with everything you eat today, always attempt to buy organic.

Canola oil contains mostly monounsaturated oils and actually contains the least amount of saturated fat of any edible oil. Better than olive for baking and cooking because is handles high temperatures better. Furthermore, you want to look for "expeller-pressed" that reasonably assures you that the oil was not extracted with the use of chemicals nor were pesticides used on the rapeseeds. Grapeseed oil is another good choice for light frying or sauteing.

Avocados have earned an undeserved reputation for being high in fat (you will note that a serving is 1/6 of an avocado), and this has caused many to shy away from what is a really healthy and enjoyable food. Avocado has a similar fat content as do almonds. The point to keep in mind is that avocados are fatty for sure, but the fat is monounsaturated fat. This is a good fat or one that is "heart-friendly", high in vitamins C and E, potassium, and folate.

Consider the example of walnuts. There was a research study that found walnuts may help to protect your arteries from high-fat meals. Even though we now know that olive oil and walnuts both protect the heart by reducing inflammation in the arteries, those eating walnuts appeared to have preserved the elasticity of the arteries, according to the Journal of the American College of Cardiology.

Flaxseed (ground) can be easily added to vegetable sautes, cereals, salads, and soups for example. Flaxseed contains omega-3s. Plant chemicals in omegas contain lignans, which are believed to have a role against cancer, especially breast cancer.

Even with healthy fats you must be very mindful of portion sizes and number of daily servings.

Code	number of daily healthy fat portions
1800	4
1600	3
1400	3
1200	3

digits 7&8

Aerobic Exercise

The 7th & 8th digits in the Diet Code always represent the (60) sixty minutes of daily aerobic exercise. The top aerobic exercise amongst weight loss superstars is walking. Twenty-eight percent of NWCR participants cite walking as their exclusive form of exercise. The key here is to find something you enjoy.

876-554-**60**83

The relevant question here is not how much exercise do you need in order to lose the weight, but, more importantly, to keep it off. Well, there are really two types of exercise that you need to understand in order to answer this question. These two are aerobic and strength training or anaerobic. Here we are concerned with aerobic exercise. This is an exercise such as walking, swimming, rowing, running, cycling, or dancing for instance intended to keep your heart rate within a certain zone.

In an effort to slow the current obesity pandemic here in the United States, the government has recently urged individuals to get 60 minutes of moderate to vigorous activity most days of the week. This is up from 30 minutes. This new standard or level, according to government experts, will allow you to manage your current weight or stop weight gain. If this level of exercise is effective, which it is, then the 46% of U.S. adults that only currently get 30 minutes each day are statistically fighting a losing battle.

All of this really begs the question versus answering the question of how much exercise is *really* required to not only lose the weight but to keep it off permanently? The real answer will likely be found not in some college lab but in the real life experiences of people who have struggled and overcome. This figure is somewhere between 60 and 90 minutes each day in order to maintain weight loss. This is based on solid research (surveys of thousands of weight loss superstars). A group of thousands of individuals who have achieved an average weight loss of around 73 pounds known as the National Weight Control Registry (NWCR) presents some of the best independent evidence. This group of researchers continually follow thousands of participants who have lost a minimum of 30 pounds and *kept it off for at least a year.*

In a survey of this group, 28% of the NWCR participants cited *walking* as their only form of physical activity. About half of the total, combined walking with some other form of planned exercise such as aerobics, biking, or swimming. Walking was, by far, the most popular form of physical activity. Not surprisingly, only 9% of registry participants reported keeping their weight off without engaging in any physical activity.

These folks are serious walkers, averaging between 11,000 and 12,000 steps per day. This is the equivalent of between 5.5 to 6 miles per day. In the final analysis, you have to get moving and stay moving in order to lose the weight and to keep it off. In terms of calorie expenditure, women expended about 2,500 k/cal/week and men, about 3,300 k/cal/week. This equates to a very high level of activity equal to 60 to 90 minutes of moderate-intensity physical activity per day.

Again, the NWCR is a significant contribution to resolving the question, but it is only a survey. In surveys, people tend to under-estimate calorie intake and to then under report. Therefore, the Diet Code has tested many of the ideas put forth by the NWCR participants.

There are additional benefits to a regular exercise program such as: strengthening of the heart, lungs, and a lowering of blood pressure. The positive effects are numerous, but I want to focus on two in particular. First, many people I have worked with have been mildly to moderately depressed in addition to being clinically obese. As a professional, I recognize just as all of you do that when you feel down and blue, you simply do not have the energy to get up to exercise. However, there is a growing mountain of evidence that strongly suggests physical activity may be very ef-fective in combating mild to moderate depression.

I work as a performance expert and life coach. Coaches listen more than talk ideally, but much of what we do with clients is communicating either directly or indirectly. Through this dialogue and when exercise is included - many clients have been able to either reduce or eliminate the need for medication. There is evidence that aerobic exercise and anaerobic exercises are equally effective for symptoms related to depression. There is evidence that exercising with a friend may be of some benefit because of the support and connection provided. My experience has been that being in a coaching relationship or in some type of sustained-partnership model is also effective for the same reasons. With respect to stress and anxiety levels, regular even brief aerobic exercise may affect your mood in a positive way. Once you begin to pay closer attention to your actual mood before and after exercise, you are likely to notice a positive consistent change.

Day of week	aerobic exercise
monday	60 minutes of aerobic exercise
tuesday	60 minutes of aerobic exercise
wednesday	60 minutes of aerobic exercise
thursday	60 minutes of aerobic exercise
friday	60 minutes of aerobic exercise
saturday	60 minutes of aerobic exercise

digit **9**

Strength training

The 9th digit in the Diet Code always represents the number of minutes you will strength or resistance train on a daily basis in order to lose and maintain your healthy weight range while building lean muscle tissue regardless of your code or stage.... Lean muscle helps increase your metabolism and you lose more weight.

876-554-60**8**3

Strength training or resistance training increases the percentage of muscle in your body. Because muscle is metabolically active tissue, the more muscular you are - the higher your metabolism will be. This, in turn, means that you will burn more calories even as you rest and ultimately you will burn more fat.

Jorge Cruise is AOL's online weight loss coach and the author of the popular *8 Minutes in the Morning* book series. The program consists of two daily exercises, six days a week. To those who may be skeptical that eight minutes a day can accomplish much, it *is* possible to reshape your body if you do the exercises with the proper intensity. This approach eliminates the commute time and the need for expensive equipment. You only need a set of dumbbells and the entire program can be done at home. Or, you can do push ups, sit ups, squats, and pull ups. And, everyone, no matter how busy has 8 minutes. Find what you enjoy and get to it.

Many clients ask the following question, "How important is exercise to weight loss?" I always find the following analogy useful in my attempt to answer the question. Just as a car runs on gas, our bodies run on the blood sugar or glucose and fat circulating in your blood. When you exercise enough to minimize the amount of blood sugar in your blood, hormones are released that instruct your fat cells to release fat into your blood. The fat is then available for muscles that need it to be used as fuel, and you end up with less fat on your body.

Exercise plays a very important role in maintaining a healthy body. However, it is a huge mistake to look to exercise as your primary weight loss tactic. For example, to lose a pound of fat, you need to burn 3,500 calories. Since walking a mile burns about 80 calories per hour, you would have to walk 44 miles to lose a single pound.

Losing weight can be much easier if you combine exercising with a little calorie cutting. If you want to lose one pound a week, then you will need to create an average 500 calorie deficit each day of the week. You can achieve this by burning off about 300 calories (in a 3 to 4 mile walk or an exercise class) and by cutting back on what you eat by 200 calories (a can of soda and a couple pats of butter) each day.

Strength training helps you prevent the loss of muscle, keeps your metabolism running at a high level, and maintain good posture. Many of my clients have the intention of losing significant amounts of weight. In order to ensure the greatest chance for that success, you must engage in some form of resistance or strength training as part of your program. Below I have included a sample training schedule for your review. The most important consideration here is to find a routine that you enjoy, which will increase the chances of you staying with the program long enough to see the results. Whatever form of resistance you decide upon - do something you enjoy.

days	8 minutes strength training activity	natural resistance	dumbbell workout
monday	chest & back		
tuesday	shoulder & abs		
wednesday	biceps & triceps		
thursday	quads & hamstrings		
friday	calves & glutes		
saturday	inner & outer thighs		

digit **10**

Autogenics

The 10th digit in the Diet Code always represents the number of Autogenic or AT daily sessions. Each day you will practice 3 visualization or stress management sessions regardless of what code or stage you find yourself. You will learn a skill that will serve you throughout your life. AT is a simple and powerful tool.

876-554-608**3**

THERE ARE SEVERAL PRECAUTIONS TO CONSIDER PRIOR TO LEARNING AUTOGENICS .

ALTHOUGH (AT) AUTOGENICS IS A RATHER SIMPLE TECHNIQUE, IT IS A VERY POWERFUL ONE. CONSEQUENTLY, IT MAY NOT BE SUITABLE FOR EVERYONE. YOU SHOULD ALWAYS LEARN THE METHOD FROM A QUALIFIED INSTRUCTOR WHENEVER POSSIBLE. AUTOGENICS SHOULD NOT BE UNDERTAKEN UNDER "ANY" OF THE FOLLOWING CIRCUMSTANCES:

1. During or immediately following a heart attack (acute myocardial infraction),

2. If you are a diabetic undergoing insulin treatment, because insulin consumption and utilization may swing wildly during AT (which results in the need for constant monitoring of both blood and urine therefore it is ill-advised for the majority of diabetics),

3. If you suffer glaucoma,

4. If you suffer from psychotic conditions such as schizophrenia or severe depression associated with hallucinations or feelings of unreality,

5. If you have had electric shock treatment,

6. If you are an active alcoholic or drug abuser,

7. If you suffer from epilepsy, or

8. If you have ever had a prolonged episode of unconsciousness,

If you do not fall into any of these categories, then there is no reason why you should not be able to begin AT at this point.

INTRODUCTION

Autogenic training or therapy, as it is known in many places around the world, is one of the most powerful and effective mind-body techniques for reducing stress and for unlocking the unlimited healing powers within each of us. In this chapter, you will learn the step-by-step process in a series of simple mental exercises. These exercises will help you to reach a deep level of relaxation.

There are several ways that Autogenics (AT) may be helpful to you in achieving your weight loss goals. First, most who struggle with weight often respond to stress triggers in their environment by overeating. Therefore, by reducing the overall level of stress, it is less likely for these to come into play. Through both AT offloading exercises and positive suggestions, the vast majority find good results in this regard.

AT has proven its effectiveness in over 3,000 published scientific studies throughout the entire world. AT has been used effectively with numerous medical conditions, used effectively by industry to reduce employee healthcare costs, and it has been an integral part of training for numerous professional and olympic champions.

Some of the additional benefits include:

. an improved ability to concentrate

. greater ability to reconcile unresolved emotions

. notable increases in energy levels

. strengthened immune response

. improved overall health

THE HISTORY OF AUTOGENICS

Autogenics, commonly known as AT, was originally developed by physician (neurologist and psychiatrist), Dr. Johannes Schultz in the beginning of the twentieth century. He went to Switzerland to study medicine in 1907 where he eventually studied psychiatry in 1909. It was at this time that he authored a review of Freud's Psychoanalysis.

During a meeting between the two men, Freud commented, "Surely you do not believe that you could heal?" Schultz replied, "By no means, but I think that, like a gardener, I could remove obstacles hindering a person's true development." Freud ended the conversation with a smile.

In 1912, Otto Binswanger invited Schultz to Jena. Schultz then succeeded Binswanger as Professor of Psychiatry in 1915. He, Schultz had been deeply influenced by the groundbreaking work of Professor Oscar Vogt (1870-1959), a brilliant psychiatrist and neuro-physiologist who had dedicated his life to psychosomatic medicine, what he referred to as the Mind-Body problem.

In his research, Vogt noticed that patients achieved a sense of well-being while practicing very simple verbal exercises in an effort to induce an altered state. Patient complaints such as headache, anxiety, fatigue tended to no longer exist. Additionally, patients noted sensations of heaviness and warmth. Schultz had wondered whether patients could reach a similar state without hypnosis, by simply directing their attention to sensations of heaviness and warmth in their limbs.

He found they were able to, under certain conditions utilizing passive concentration and employing simple verbal formulas, produce heaviness and warmth. In 1912, Schultz published Autogenic Organ Exercises. By 1924, he had moved to Berlin to be more closely aligned with Vogt who was conducting research at the Neuro-Biological Institute for Brain Research. Schultz also continued his own personal research, in 1932 he published his first edition of Autogenic Therapy. In this masterwork, he details the clinical application of the six standard AT formulas. These six represent the core of the AT program you are about to learn.

In the late 1940s, Dr. Wolfgang Luthe, began to study psychosomatic medicine and Autogenic Therapy with Schultz. In the 1950's, Luthe emigrated to Montreal, Canada. There he continued to develop AT as Assistant Professor of Psychophysiology at the University of Montreal. The two men worked together conducting research into all areas of AT. In 1969, they published five volumes of AT. These have now been published in nine languages. Schultz died in 1970. The volumes still stand as a major work in the area.

In 1978, Dr. Malcolm Carruthers, a British physician, and psychotherapist, Vera Diamond went to study AT under Luthe in Montreal and later introduced the method in London. They later helped to establish what is now known as the British Autogenic Society in 1984. AT is now practiced widely throughout Europe and in Japan. Institutions such as the Schultz Institute in Berlin and the Oscar Vogt Institute at Kyushu University in Japan are preeminent in the field of AT research, development, and training. AT is currently used as a tool in addition to allopathic approaches in the N.H.S. in the U.K.

I have been studying and practicing AT since 1999. In 2004, I began formal study with the famed psychotherapist, Vera Diamond in London and was her last student prior to her death in 2005.

THE PROCESS OF AT

Clients usually learn AT over a period of several weeks. During this time, AT becomes part of an overall lifestyle. Clients note a number of changes toward greater emotional stability, a reduction in stress and anxiety, and increases in overall well-being and health.

All of these reports are supported by studies into the physiological changes that come along with the regular use of AT. At the core of these positive changes is passive concentration, which is a detached yet alert state of mind where AT exercises are conducted.

In the modern world, we live much of our lives in the left hemisphere of our brains. This is the center of logic, language, planning, and analysis. In our day-to-day experience we are in what seems to be a constant struggle to achieve, to reach the next goal, to make the next meeting or deadline. The stresses of modern life exist like never before.

All of these combined pressures lead to anxiety, frustration, feelings of failure, and an overall feeling that life is somehow out of control and we are therefore powerless in the face of events that seem to be beyond our influence.

Through this process of viewing our lives as a series of obstacles, we can become numb to the warning signs from our bodies and to our intuitions from our greater wisdom, our unconscious. Furthermore, we often become desensitized to the emotional needs of those close to us. Too often the broader meaning of life is lost. In the process we can become reactionary.

FIGHT OR FLIGHT

This obliviousness to the more meaningful aspects of life is further exacerbated by the way that too many of us respond to these challenges of modern pressures and life. We are actually programmed to respond in this manner. This idea is based on an ancient physiological response to *any* perceived threat. Then, it was the saber-toothed tiger, but now it could be an unreasonable deadline, or our perception of a 'reasonable' deadline as unreasonable, or when a tyrant boss simply enters the room.

This fight or flight response produces the same physiological response in all humans; pupils dilate, heartbeat increases, adrenaline is released, gastric activity decreases, the bronchi of the lungs dilate, and muscular strength increases. All of this occurs instantaneously and lasts for a short period of time.

Once the crisis or danger has passed, the autonomic nervous system will eventually switch back to a state of rest and relaxation. Predictably; pupils will contract, heartbeat will return to normal rate, and digestion will resume. It is not difficult to understand how this system has served us well throughout our history.

However, in our modern lives, we are constantly exposed to challenges that do not result in a need for a burst of physical energy, and that do not diminish in a short time period. For instance, living under a constant threat of an impending layoff in an uncertain economy or awaiting medical test results, which may require weeks to confirm. Situations such as these can and do drag on sometimes for weeks, months, or even years.

Therefore, with a perceived threat at the office or in a relationship or at home, we tend to handle these quite differently than say an oncoming vicious dog. We do not run away from the threat in the office or the threat to our relationship do we? On the contrary, we often allow them to simply simmer. We often hear, "Go for a walk," or "Just let it go." On a conscious level, all of us understand this, but on a biological level it is never that straightforward.

Our bodies can't distinguish perceived threats from real threats. Our understanding of language provides us with the tools and the ability to predict threats that are often abstract in nature, to imagine the outcome of these predictions, and to react to our own imagination as if it were real. When you take the family pet in for a critical x-ray or test, Fluffy has none of the same anticipatory fear or anxiety as we might experience in a comparable situation. In our case, our imagination and our ability to think come into play whereas Fluffy *appears* just happy to be in a new surrounding.

This is why AT can be such an important tool for us. It enables you to shift into a rest and relaxation state at will. The enhanced coping effects along with the regular practice of AT and passive concentration encourage this shift to a different mode of perception, away from judging or striving toward witnessing. For many, this may be a novel experience, and may require the personalized support of a trained professional. However, you, perhaps like me initially, may be able to gain a tremendous amount of self-insight through deep introspection. Remember, there are no right or wrong answers in this process. You only need to remain fully present for the process.

Clients regularly report the following: a greater toughness in response to emotional and physical upsets; a freedom from unwanted habits; greater spontaneity in relationships; a freedom from anxiety; a calm center with themselves; and a restoration of a sense of control in their lives.

Furthermore, they report an increase in creativity and openness to intuition. You may booomo moro awaro of omotiono, feelingo, and memories, including disturbing ones that may have been repressed for some time. This expanded access to feelings, memories, intuition, and creativity are all associated with right-brain activities. Analysis of the central nervous system has shown an increased balance between the two hemispheres along with an increase in Alpha wave activity and an upward shift into the Theta region. Physiological tests further support reports of reduced stress by users of AT along with measured reductions in blood pressure and stress hormones.

THEORY AND RATIONALE

All of us, from time to time, repress emotions related to negative experiences such as anger, guilt, rage, resentment, and sadness. This inability to deal with or to reconcile this emotional material is the source of much unhappiness and even disease. AT helps you to get in touch with the true emotional nature of your feelings. More importantly, AT provides a tool to *discharge these emotions safely and satisfactorily through specific controlled exercises,* rather than repressing and storing them.

Through this process of self-regulation, healing, and adjustment that takes place during the practice of AT, you are able to find your true center. In the midst of this progressive process, the mind/body seems to rid itself of not only present but also past stresses, memories, and emotions that are yet to be resolved. This process of re-lease known as "autogenic discharge," usually takes the form of brief and sporadic muscle twitches or as an awareness of unrecognized feelings. These brief yet harmless muscle releases are a very important part of the process of throwing off life's stresses and old baggage.

AT does not "paper over" issues, you rather become acutely aware of them thereby ensuring that the gains you earn will be permanent and not fleeting. The process of AT is analogous to peeling the layers of an onion where each layer might be an emotion, a feeling, memory or experience. As you move to deeper and deeper levels, invariably you engage potentially more difficult emotional material. The process quite often results in personal growth, self-development, and in a more positive feeling about your life and your prospects as a human being.

THREE GOLDEN RULES OF AT

These (3) three rules must always be observed when doing AT.

1. CANCEL IMMEDIATELY if you get into touch with any particularly uncomfortable feelings or sensations during an exercise.

2. CANCEL IMMEDIATELY if you begin to see concrete images, such as a duck floating across a pond. If you do see such an image, <u>DO NOT dwell on it no matter how pleasant the image may be as this may lead to the *sudden* release of unconscious material.</u> This is not desirable at this point in your AT experience.

3. NEVER CHANGE OR ALTER AN EXERCISE FORMULA WITHOUT THE SPECIFIC GUIDANCE OF YOUR INSTRUCTOR. Close to a century of research and clinical practice have gone into the design of each to produce these safe and effective formulas. You must heed this warning. There may be cases where a formula may need to be either modified or omitted; however, that decision must be made in conjunction with a qualified trainer or you must follow the guidelines specified here in the event that no such trainer is available.

EXERCISE POSITIONS

There are four (4) skills you must grasp prior to beginning the actual AT exercises. These are: 1) Exercise positions, 2) Scanning, 3) Passive concentration, and 4) Canceling. We begin with the three exercise positions.

One of the most important considerations in understanding exercises is that each of the three positions must be *comfortable* prior to your beginning each of the exercises. In addition to your comfort, you should ensure:

. your bladder and bowels are empty,

. your shoes are removed and any tight clothing is loosened,

. your physical practice area is comfortable, dimly lit, quiet, and as isolated as possible, especially during the *initial* stages of AT, and

. finally, during the day's practice each of the three positions are utilized.

Lying Position

Your arms should lie flat beside your body, slightly bent at the elbows, and the palms of the hands placed flat on the surface of the couch or mattress. The tips of your feet falling slightly to the outside. I find that it is easier to begin practicing with this position for most people.

The lying position has several advantages. I will often complete my first daily exercise before even officially rising in the morning. You may find this to be a great way to start your day. Again physical comfort must be your top priority as it is impossible to relax if you are not comfortable.

Seated Position

This position allows you to use an executive office type chair with a high back and arm rests or a recliner that provides both neck and arm support. Your elbows should be kept at an almost right angle allowing your arm muscles to remain in a balanced and relaxed position. Your feet should be allowed to fall slightly to the outside - thereby avoiding muscular tension in your thigh muscles (most people unconsciously close their knees while seated).

Rag-doll Position

This position is for use on a bench or a chair without proper neck and arm support. There will times when neither of the two previous positions is practical or available to you. When this occurs, you will be able to use this position, known as the "rag-doll" position.

In this position, allow your head to sink into your chest (it is important to note that your head should be in alignment with your spine). Also, allow your arms to hang at your sides *or* your forearms, close to the elbow, may rest comfortably on your thighs, if you find this more comfortable.

In this vertically-oriented position, there should be almost no muscular activity or tension because the skeleton is being held by the spine and its tendons. Each AT position is designed to minimize muscular tension while increasing your physical comfort. It is very important to note that each of these three positions should be mastered prior to moving onto the next stage, scanning.

SCANNING

After entering an AT position, next you *always* scan prior to doing an actual exercise. Scanning is a step-by-step process where you will "check in" with different parts of your body. In effect, seeing how each part of your physical body is doing by briefly focusing on specific parts. You may find it helpful to focus your attention mentally on each part as you briefly scan that particular area.

Far too many of us only become aware of our bodies when some part of it either breaks down or sends a signal such as pain or distress.

There are two primary reasons for scanning:

1) to center yourself before beginning an AT exercise, and

2) to get in touch with your body and possible areas of tension before beginning the actual exercise.

The actual scanning process is as follows:

Your eyes should already be closed. Take your mind to the tips of your toes moving upward from each foot simultaneously. Then mentally continue upward to your heels, to your ankles, calves, shins, thighs, hips, and pelvic area, stomach, chest, shoulders, upper arms, elbows, forearms, wrists, hands, and to the fingertips of each hand.

Now, take your mind to your back beginning with your buttocks area, up to the large muscles of your back, around your shoulder blades, up the back of your neck, over the scalp, the forehead, around your eyes, your cheeks, the jaw, which should sag or hang loosely and comfortably in a relaxed position. If you should find it difficult to get in touch with a specific part, as some do, here are two options available to you.

1. While completing the scan, with your eyes closed run your dominant hand lightly over that specific area of your body in an effort to get in touch with that area.

2. Or, you may imagine that you are giving yourself a massage in the affected area(s). Some imagine painting the affected area with a large paintbrush. Be creative. You are only limited by your own imagination.

Many find they tend to scan rather slowly initially, but eventually it will only require a few seconds. Speed is not ever a concern in AT; however, as you progress, you will be able to go through the full exercise in a very short length of time. The important points to keep in mind with respect to scanning are to 1) always use the same exact routine each time you scan, and 2) to get in touch with all parts of your body as you scan. Next, passive concentration.

PASSIVE CONCENTRATION

Passive concentration is *the most* important aspect of learning AT and may be the most challenging to grasp, especially for those of us in the West. Passive concentration although simple in theory, can be challenging in practice. It is not uncommon for some clients to experience difficulty in achieving passive concentration for the first three to four weeks of AT practice. I personally had tremendous difficulty initially. You, however, may have no difficulty at all.

Many of us have been taught or trained to concentrate hard and to make things happen by pressing for an outcome or a result. Many of us grow up believing that the harder we work, the hard we concentrate, the more likely we are to achieve our goals. This is the exact opposite of passive concentration.

In passive concentration, you are <u>not trying to do anything, or achieve anything, or reach any outcome.</u> All you are doing is sitting back and simply observing what is happening in your body and your mind as you go through the AT exercise and formulas. Next, canceling.

CANCELING

At the conclusion of every AT exercise, you end each in the same exact manner, by canceling the exercise. In AT, canceling is very important. Canceling is a technique that allows you to return to your normal awareness and reflexes. You should practice canceling several times prior to beginning regular AT exercises.

Canceling involves four (4) distinct steps.

1) Clenching and releasing both fists tightly a few times

2) Bending your elbows briskly and inwardly and stretching your arms back outward or downward four times (as if you were performing a very quick series of (4) four dumbbell curls)

3) Taking a deep breath in and holding it, and

4) Opening your eyes and then breathing out.

Note: It is *critically important* for you to open your eyes just before exhaling. If not, the cancelation may not be fully effective. Again, you simply need to open your eyes just before exhalation to properly cancel. You can actually cancel as many times as you like. The point is to ensure that you have completely left an AT state.

Having now been exposed to:

a) AT positions
b) Scanning
c) Passive Concentration, and
d) Canceling... you are now ready to begin the first standard AT exercise. Good luck, relax, enjoy yourself, and remember to be kind to yourself through this process.

EXERCISE ONE

HEAVY LIMBS

Exercise one is divided into three (3) sections: day 1, days 2-4, and days 5-7. Most clients learn this initial lesson over the course of a seven day cycle over one to two weeks. This first exercise is very simple to learn yet it is very important and will provide several benefits as you progress through the remaining exercises. For example:

. your concentration is likely to improve as a result

. it will enable you to practice when you are short on time

. it can be used when you are angry, feeling emotional, or when it is not possible to complete a full-length exercise

. it can be used throughout the day to reinforce learnings as you progress deeper into the exercises.

Exercise one, heavy limbs, begins by focusing on your musculature, in part because your muscles are the easiest to influence through conscious efforts. Muscular relaxation has been well-documented and can be achieved quickly through hypnotic techniques for example.

We actually experience muscle relaxation as "heaviness" in our extremities. For instance, it is likely that you have experienced a limb that seemed to have been detached (where your arm has "fallen asleep" and feels heavy, almost detached).

On the other hand, whenever you focus your attention on *any* external stimulus, this results in muscular tension. For instance, whenever you look, speak, or reach for anything, you produce muscular tension. It is a well known scientific fact that even when you imagine a physical movement, such as, shooting a free throw, your muscles make the same exact movements as they would during an actual shot. Consider the implications. That is, each intention or imagining of an action will result in movement in that direction. For example, you can imagine your way to anything, better eating habits or a more consistent habit of regular exercise.

Exercise number one begins by focusing on your dominant arm and continues until the sensation of heaviness begins to generalize or spread to your other limbs. This is possible because all of our limbs are connected by the nervous system. The two things that will dictate your success above all else will be your consistency in practicing each day and your intention. Be diligent in both.

Be mindful of passive concentration? This process is not about striving, pressing, or trying too hard. Don't force anything here. Just sit back and notice what is happening. For many, the feeling of pronounced heaviness may begin to occur more rapidly between days four to six.

With almost a century of clinical experience, every clinician will tell you of the gap between theory and practice. The point here is that unexpected things will occur, family and work obligations will continue to be a reality, things will arise that will present challenges to your regular practice. Stay focused on what you want versus the obstacles.

I want to provide you advance notice of what may be possible challenges during exercise one. It is quite natural that whenever you experience new sensations they are often experienced as "different" or "strange." Many of these are normal correlates to muscular and vascular relaxation and yet puzzling and may even result in initial though brief anxiety in some.

Rest assured that these are completely normal and are experienced by many. For instance, these may include: brief localized muscle spasms, tingling, numbness, a pulling sensation, perceived swelling in the fingers, and/or a sense of detachment of a limb. Some may not experience any of these. If you do experience cramping, you are quite often trying too hard to *produce* a result, which ironically results in you being less likely to achieve the desired results.

EXERCISE ONE

DAY 1

1. AT Position

2. Scan (with eyes closed)

3. Mentally connect with your *dominant* arm, which runs from your shoulder to your fingertips.

4. Repeat the following formula sub-vocally, to yourself, three (3) times:

"MY RIGHT (LEFT) ARM IS HEAVY." X 3

5. Cancel

6. Repeat the entire procedure two more times (excluding the scan) for a total of three times, provided you had a pleasant experience. Be sure to note each experience in your training notebook.

7. Throughout this entire training, the schedule is 3 X 3, which means you will complete three complete sets of the exercise at three different times during each day until instructed otherwise.

EXERCISE ONE

DAYS 2-4

1. AT position

2. Scan (with eyes closed)

3. Mentally connect with your dominant arm (from your shoulder to fingertips)

4. Repeat the following phrases sub-vocally, to yourself, three (3) times each passively while observing what happens:

"MY RIGHT (LEFT) ARE IS HEAVY." X 3

"MY LEFT (RIGHT) ARM IS HEAVY." X 3

"MY ARMS ARE HEAVY." X 3

5. Cancel

6. Repeat the entire procedure two (2) more times (excluding the scan) for a total of three times [3x3 training schedule]. Note your experiences in your training notebooks.

EXERCISE ONE

DAYS 5-7 (HEAVY ARMS & LEGS)

1. AT position

2. Scan (with eyes closed)

3. Mentally connect with your dominant arm once again (from shoulder to fingertips)

4. Repeat the following sub-vocally, to yourself, three (3) times each:

<blockquote>

"MY RIGHT (LEFT) ARM IS HEAVY." X 3

"MY LEFT (RIGHT) ARM IS HEAVY." X 3

"MY ARMS ARE HEAVY." X 3

"MY RIGHT (LEFT) LEG IS HEAVY." X 3

"MY LEFT (RIGHT) LEG IS HEAVY." X 3

"MY LEGS ARE HEAVY." X 3

"MY ARMS AND LEGS ARE HEAVY." X 3

</blockquote>

5. Cancel

6. Repeat the entire procedure twice more for a total of three (3) times, excluding the scan between cancellations. Note your experience afterwards. Cancel immediately if you see concrete images or experience unpleasant sensations. Remember the 3x3 training schedule. If you are able after day seven to experience heaviness in your arms and legs after a brief moment of inner concentration,

you are ready to move onto the next exercise. If you are not able, spend another week on exercise one prior to moving onto the second exercise. Remember this is not a race. Take your time and be patient with yourself.

HEAVY NECK AND SHOULDERS

During the first exercise, you may have found some difficulty in concentrating during the latter part of the week, days five through seven. This is a common experience. Also during this past week, you may have experienced your eyelids flickering along with the possibility of having difficulty in keeping your eyes closed. Again, these are normal reactions commonly experienced.

These responses are mainly due to not being prepared or ready to "let go" and completely relax. Respect this reluctance to "let go" as it may be your unconscious attempt to protect you from going too far - too fast. It is designed to protect us. The fear of loss of control is powerful in all of us.

The other consideration that you may have noticed from this past week is likely to relate to your awareness of external distractions. For instance, you may begin to notice small things all around you that may have gone unnoticed before. AT is partly about raising your awareness on multiple levels. Consider your body. Since your body is not able to verbally speak directly to you, then it attempts to communicate in different ways in an effort to focus your attention. Be patient and kind to yourself throughout this process.

In the end, you will find some exercises result in a noticeably deeper level of relaxation than do some others. Relax and enjoy this great experience.

During this week's exercise, there are two versions to be learned: a standard version and an abbreviated version, to be used during the course of the day, especially when you are short on time.

In exercise (2) two, heavy neck and shoulders, you will be concentrating on experiencing <u>the feeling of heaviness in the muscles of your neck and shoulders.</u> As you might imagine, we tend to carry large amounts of tension in these areas along with huge amounts of stored tension and repressed emotional material.

We tend not to pay that much attention to these areas, in part I suspect, because of their physical location and the relative difficulty of reaching them. Nonetheless, I think it is useful to describe, in detail, the area I wish you to focus your attention.

Your neck and shoulder muscles include a large sheet of neck muscles that lie over the back muscles at the top of your spine. These begin at the base of your skull and run down and out over your shoulders, creating a triangle extending down into the middle of your back. If you were to imagine a diamond shaped area, this area would be similar in shape.

Also, there are two very large groups of back muscles that run downward along each side of your spine in a series of cords. These run from your buttocks upward to the base of your skull. As you might imagine, when these go into spasm or become tense, you often experience a severe neck ache, head ache, back ache or all three simultaneously.

EXERCISE TWO

DAYS 1-7

1. AT position

2. Scan

3. Mentally connect to your *dominant* arm (right or left), and become a passive observer of yourself and see what happens as you go through the following formula sub-vocally, to yourself:

"MY RIGHT (LEFT) ARM IS HEAVY"

"MY ARMS & LEGS ARE HEAVY" X 3

"MY NECK & SHOULDERS ARE HEAVY" X 3

"I AM AT PEACE" X 3

4. Cancel

5. Repeat this entire procedure two more times (excluding the scan in between exercises).

6. Repeat the whole exercise 3 complete times each day (3x3), using a different position each time.

THE SHORT EXERCISE

(use when you can not complete the full version)

In those situations where practicing the full version of the exercise is not possible or is impractical, consider using this "short" or "partial" exercise. You simply are going to repeat the following sentence sub-vocally from 70 to 100 times, always sub-vocally or to yourself, the formula,

"MY NECK & SHOULDERS ARE HEAVY."

There are a few very important differences in using the "Short Exercise".....

.DO NOT take you mind to your neck and shoulders

. DO NOT close your eyes

. DO NOT get into an AT position

. DO NOT add the phrase, "I am at peace."

EXERCISE THREE

WARMTH

This week's exercise involves experiencing the sensation of warmth. Consequently, it is important to note that any procedure that involves the dilation of blood vessels is not without risk since any change in blood distribution affects the entire system. The exercise should be completed or attempted only by those for whom no **vascular** risks are known to exist. As always, I will now attempt to alert you to some of the predictable yet novel experiences you *may* encounter in this warmth exercise, known as vasodilation.

Some client's experience challenges in one of two extremes, while some experience none. Some experience a cooling of the arm while others have reported a burning sensation in their arm. Both of these usually completely disappear with continued usage.

If however, the discomfort of either cooling or of a burning sensation continues where either makes it consistently uncomfortable to use the formula, then you should, as always, cancel immediately. The other alternative in this instance is to alter the formula to, "My arm is pleasantly warm," versus, "warm."

You may also notice an inner, flowing sensation of warmth observed very quickly in the elbow and lower arm.

Just as you experienced heaviness associated with muscular relaxation, the experience of warmth has been well documented at more than 1 degree celsius and a 6-8 C increase in tissue warmth in highly trained persons.

Experiencing the sensation of warmth in your limbs is this exercise's focus. Each exercise is progressive in that it will build on the skill you learned in the previous one. Each will also follow a normal sequence of physiological changes that are correlated with relaxation. In this instance, as your muscles relax, the blood vessels open and the circulation to a given area increases. You will likely experience an increased sensation of warmth in that area. As blood flow increases to a specific area, you may also experience a throbbing or pulsing sensation in that area.

Again, this can be unsettling for some, but be assured that there is no cause for fear or anxiety. I should point out that 30 to 40 % of AT clients may never experience one or more of the sensations they are focusing on in a particular exercise. The more important point here is to stay on the path and to see the process through to the end independent of any particular physiological response or lack thereof.

You have very likely experienced brief muscle twitches during AT practice. This is your body's attempt to release stress. You may find some of the later offloading exercises very useful in this regard, the motor loosening exercise in particular may be useful.

Changes in emotional activity are also associated with changes in blood flow. For example, consider what occurs when a person blushes. Even a small change such as this affects the entire cardiovascular system including arteries, capillaries to the organs, venous blood flow, and flow through the skin and muscles.

The distribution of blood is regulated by dilation and constriction in response to changes in your nervous system and variables such as physical activity, general state of arousal, and inhibition.

One of the most important considerations to keep in mind is to *passively observe* the feelings or sensations you are experiencing, while never attempting to influence what is happening,

While the intended direction is for many to experience warmth, you may also experience coolness or even a feeling of coldness. This could be due to a cool or cold room or if you carry negative emotions or memories at the limb level, the most superficial level at which we can experience unresolved tension.

On the other hand, you may be more acutely aware of emotions such as anger or anxiety. This may present itself as an over-expression of the emotion or in a far less obvious manner such as difficulty in concentrating, greater irritability, increased neck pain or pain in other areas most especially during AT practice. You may again notice muscle twitches not only during AT but also while you sleep. This may indicate your being in contact with unresolved or repressed past stress or emotional material.

This point is especially relevant at this junction because many clients experience a "rough spot" between the 3rd and the 5th exercises of AT practice. Of course everyone will have a unique experience; however, many people generally have a smooth start (during exercise one to three), then a more difficult period (exercise three through five), and then a smoother final period (exercise 6 through completion).

We all have unique "luggage" or life experiences that shape us and reflect our different stages of incompleteness. This is why the offloading exercises are so important as they provide another opportunity to release unresolved issues. AT provides an opportunity to reconcile unresolved pain or trauma from an injury. Through offloading, chronicling your experience in your notebook, or through autogenic discharge you may find that by giving a voice to the experience, you may be able to release it.

You will find learning this exercise to be similar in some ways to the heaviness exercise as you will learn each limb separately. There are a few additional changes in the formula. For example, this "warmth" formula is to be introduced between "heaviness" and "heavy shoulders", which will now be used as a type of book-end (to be placed at the end of the exercise) in the formula going forward.

At the point where you are able to produce warmth in your dominant arm and later in all four of your extremities, you are ready to move onto the next exercise. You may even experience warmth and heaviness that generalizes to your entire body.

EXERCISE THREE

WARMTH EXERCISE

DAYS 1-3

1. AT position

2. Scan

3. Repeat the formula:

"MY RIGHT (LEFT) ARM IS HEAVY."

"MY ARMS & LEGS ARE HEAVY." X 3

"MY RIGHT (LEFT) ARM IS WARM X 3

"MY LEFT (RIGHT) ARM IS WARM." X 3

"MY ARMS ARE WARM." X 3

"MY NECK & SHOULDERS ARE HEAVY" X 3

"I AM AT PEACE." X 3

4. Cancel

5. Repeat this entire procedure two additional times now, at least three time per day in different positions (3x3). Note your experiences in your training notebook after your session.

EXERCISE THREE

WARMTH EXERCISE (days 4-7)

1. AT position

2. Scan

3. Repeat formula:

"MY RIGHT (LEFT) ARM IS HEAVY."

"MY ARMS & LEGS ARE HEAVY." X 3

"MY RIGHT (LEFT) LEG IS WARM." X 3

"MY LEFT (RIGHT) LEG IS WARM." X 3

"MY ARMS ARE WARM." X 3

"MY RIGHT (LEFT) LEG IS WARM." X 3

"MY LEFT (RIGHT) LEG IS WARM." X 3

"MY LEGS ARE WARM." X 3

"MY ARMS & LEGS ARE WARM." X 3

"MY NECK & SHOULDERS ARE HEAVY." X 3

"I AM AT PEACE." X 3

4. Cancel and repeat two additional times, excluding the scan. Repeat entire procedure three times each day in different positions (3x3). Note your experiences. Use the short exercise if you are short on time.

EXERCISE FOUR

HEARTBEAT EXERCISE

Outside of danger, illness, injury, excitement, or fear, most do not give much thought to their heart. If you take a moment to focus on it, you may be able to perceive a faint beating sensation. Your heart, approximately the size of your fist, physically located in the lower part of your chest, its right edge is along the right side of your sternum or breast bone and its tip, in males, about at the level of the nipple (in females, at the corresponding point) - is an amazing pumping muscle.

An incredibly powerful twisting and churning muscle that works continually with only very brief relaxation periods. Its precise rhythm is regulated by the nervous system. Through learning the process of warmth you have already acquired the skill to influence the entire system through your blood vessels. You have also learned relaxation of your muscles through concentrating on the experience of heaviness. This exercise will be similar in this regard.

This exercise is the heartbeat exercise. At this point in the progression of your training, you are likely to have come into contact with feelings or emotional material that require closer attention. The heart level of experience is home to more significant emotional material. In other words, you are moving closer to the "heart" of the matter. I want to again stress the importance of 'dealing with' this through offloading exercises.

It is advisable that you *study and use this heartbeat exercise along with the next section, offloading.* There are many reasons for this; however, chief among them is that many of you will experience some difficulty in concentrating during exercises, although it is entirely possible that you may have had very little difficulty up to this point.

It is at this juncture that I feel it important to underscore the fact that all of us have a natural built-in resistance to change, even positive change. We are really designed to maintain the status quo, which is one of the reasons even minor changes are so difficult for many. This will of course require you to continue to be diligent in both your practice and your focus in order to break through this resistance to changes you are making in your life.

Because so few of us focus so little of our attention on our heart, it is a very new idea for most. Therefore, given the heart's importance to life itself, I will point out what challenges you may experience during this heartbeat exercise.

First, you should know that you can and may experience your heartbeat in any number of places on your body such as: feet, earlobes, temples, finger tips, wrist, or neck to name a few.

I recall the first time I experienced my heartbeat in my chest during an AT exercise, it was shocking and actually caused me some anxiety precisely because I was not prepared nor familiar with the experience. I have never had any personal heart problems, but family members have. Consequently, my previously unrecognized latent fear related to my own mortality arouse during this exercise and contributed to some anxious moments even though I knew what was going to occur. The point of this is that if you have any such concerns, take your time and listen to your body.

If, on the initial awareness of your heartbeat, you find it to be too distressing or uncomfortable, you can either reduce the number of repetitions in the formula or eliminate it completely. This will have no bearing on your overall experience.

EXERCISE FOUR

HEARTBEAT (DAYS 1-7)

1. AT position

2. Scan

3. Direct you attention to your dominant arm, then simply become a passive observer of your body and notice what happens as you go through the following formula:

"MY RIGHT (LEFT) ARM IS HEAVY."

"MY ARMS & LEGS ARE HEAVY & WARM." X 3

"MY HEARTBEAT IS CALM & REGULAR." X 3

"MY NECK & SHOULDERS ARE HEAVY." X 3

"I AM AT PEACE." X 3

4. Repeat the formula two additional times now (excluding the scan) and two more times throughout the day (3x3). Use different AT positions each time. Briefly note your experiences in your training notebook.

Note: If you ever experience strong, uncomfortable feelings or emotions, see concrete images, CANCEL IMMEDIATELY and return to the exercise at some later time.

OFFLOADING EXERCISES

For many of us, a big challenge exists in our ability to allow ourselves to get in touch with our positive emotions such as; love or joy, or our negative emotions such as; anger, rage, guilt, resentment, or sadness. Even when we allow ourselves to get in touch with these emotions, rarely do we allow ourselves the luxury of fully expressing them.

Repression of this unresolved emotional material runs rampant in our society. What results is a storehouse of emotional material impacting both our physical and emotional outlook and well-being. The world becomes a more gloomy place than it need be. One that is far less colorful than it has to be without free access to our full emotional range. This inability to reconcile these negative emotional states exposes us to a host of ailments, diseases, and emotional pain and suffering.

It is crucial that we become aware of and get in touch with our deep feelings and that we then employ techniques to rid ourselves of them. By releasing these stored experiences we are able to convert their tremendous negative energy into positive energy. For example, we know that the human immune system is strengthen by laughter even in the face of life-threatening illness and disease.

In AT, *offloading exercises* provide a very important tool for you to externalize these normal emotions. The exercises themselves are a critically important part of the overall process. Whenever you 'get in touch' with emotions such as; fear, resentment, rage, guilt, grief, loneliness or any number of these emotions you should use one of the offloading exercises. By continuing to ignore or dismiss them, the lingering feeling and their control over your feelings and your life will not simply evaporate.

There are distinct categories for offloading that are specifically intended to address certain emotional states. However, all of our emotions are neuro-chemically interlinked and may easily move from one to another. Consequently, it is a very good idea to experience each of the offloading exercises at some point. But for now, let us begin with the *anger* offloading exercises as we all experience this powerful emotion from time to time.

Offloading exercises are known as *intentional exercises.* Unlike the six standard AT exercises where you use passive concentration, intentional or offloading exercises are practiced with specific intent. That is, you _are_ attempting to make something occur or happen, such as offloading anger, frustration, or sadness.

Anger and Aggression Offloading

Anger, as you know, is a very powerful emotion, and repressing it requires a large amount of energy. Therefore, if you are successful in ridding yourself of anger, the net effect will be an amount of energy available to you for more productive pursuits.

Anger, not unlike sadness, is amongst the most basic of all human emotions. Through social conditioning, however, we learn that the outward expression of anger is not socially acceptable. We are conditioned to be fearful in the face of displays of anger. This along with gender conditioning makes it even more difficult for women to openly express anger, which is somehow typically considered a "male" behavioral expression.

After years of this type conditioning geared towards suppression and away from authentic emotional expression, many believe that it is somehow wrong to express anger. Certainly by adulthood most of us clearly understand the social and economic costs in such expression. What results is large numbers of people walking around as 'human time-bombs.' As too often happens, the fuse burns down resulting in nervous breakdown, stroke, heart attack, high blood pressure, chronic illness, some form of emotional meltdown, or simply consistently fewer good choices in life.

Some have repressed their anger to such an extent that they are unable to recognize, much less, fully express anger in a situation where it might be appropriate. As you might imagine, this can lead to a host of somatic illnesses such as: cancer, severe depression, backache, neck ache, or joint pain to name a few. Over time, this can also lead to feelings of great anxiety or guilt.

It is quite common to hear clients report increased irritability, either between sessions or during an AT exercise. Some clients complain of pain in the left chest area, often sharp and short-term.

As always, if any physical symptom persists, you should immediately consult your physician to determine whether there is any underlying organic cause.

When was the last time you gave yourself permission to be angry or to cry or both? I am quite often surprised when I pose this question to my clients. If you think about why tears and tear ducts were supplied in the first place, then it makes perfect sense. That is, to release emotions, as an outlet for offloading or releasing emotions such as sadness. I should point out that being angry is not a pre-condition for offloading anger. I have and continue to use it when I am in a very pleasant frame of mind.

It is, however, a good idea to create a written list in your notebook of the things that have angered you, large and small. I have seen lists that include: God, mates, partners, bosses, teachers, lovers, doctors, lawyers, or even yourself. Yes, we are quite often at the root of our own problems, and we sometimes have a tendency to blame everyone but ourselves. Begin, by always looking inward. Dr. Albert Ellis argues that it is not outside or external events or people that upset us - we upset ourselves by our thinking. The problems often reside in our interpretation of events.

The 4 Rules Must Always Be Observed When Offloading:

1. NEVER DO AN OFFLOADING EXERCISE IN AN AT POSITION!

2. NEVER OFFLOAD PRIOR TO BEDTIME.

3. NEVER OFFLOAD WITHIN ONE (1) HOUR OF AN AT EXERCISE (although offloading afterwards, even immediately is encouraged especially when having been in touch with uncomfortable material). REMEMBER TO ALWAYS CANCEL THE EXERCISE PRIOR TO OFFLOADING.

4. NEVER OFFLOAD WHEN SHORT ON TIME.

ANGER OFFLOADING EXERCISES

Snapping the Branch #1

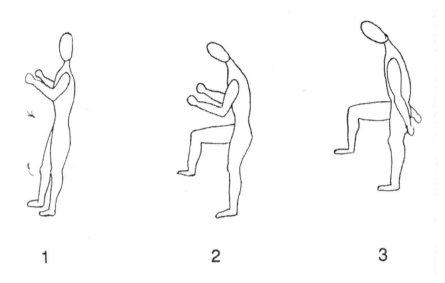

1. Stand up with your elbows bent, arms raised in front of you (as if you were about to break a twig over your knee), gather your thoughts of perhaps something or someone from your "anger" list or something that produces fear in you, or fear itself.

2. Forcefully bring your arms down, straightening your elbows and **grunting as loudly as you can.**

3. As you bring your arms down, bring one knee up at the same time as if snapping a twig over that knee. Imagine breaking the source of fear or anger over your knee. The more graphic and vivid your imagination here, the more effectively the anger or fear will be neutralized. Repeat this ten (10) times on each knee. You may feel relieved afterwards, be sure to note your feelings and experience in your notebook.

Anger Offloading Exercise #2

1. Sit forward in your chair with your forearms on your thighs.

2. Close your eyes.

3. With your palms turned up, gently tap your forearms and hands against your thighs, while <u>grunting</u> as you tap.

4. Make the tapping firmer and the grunts louder as you allow your feelings to flow out.

5. Continue until you feel "empty" of the feeling or until you feel tired.

Anger Offloading Exercise #3

1. Sit, stand, or stomp around.

2. Think of something or someone on your list. Or, you can select what you are angry about at the moment.

3. Have a passionate one-sided argument, imagine the other person is actually in the room with you and can hear you. Get in their face, if you like. Let them really hear it! Curse them, use colorful language if you feel like it. The stronger the emotions and language, the more quickly the source of your anger will likely be neutralized.

Anger Offloading Exercise #4

1. Sit forward in your chair, with a cushion in your lap.

2. Think of someone on your "anger list" and imagine placing that person into the cushion.

3. Verbally say all the thoughts or words that come into your mind. Really allow your feelings to come out.

4. Beat the cushion with your hands and fists. Stomp your feet. Do whatever you feel.

5. Continue until you either tire or feel empty of the anger.

FRUSTRATION OFFLOADING EXERCISES

The Screaming Exercise

This is one of the simplest exercises for offloading feelings of *frustration, anger, tension, etc.* When you feel like screaming at the top of your lungs, when you feel awful, but don't quite seem to know what the problem is this is a great offloading exercise to explore. You will obviously need a private space to do this exercise.

If you do not have immediate access to a private space, here is an alternative.

1. To begin, sit with a large pillow in your lap.

2. Then, take a deep breath in and scream from as deep *in the pit of your stomach* as you can into the pillow.

3. Repeat this process repeatedly until you feel empty or tired.

The Tantrum Exercise

This is another offloading exercise that provides you with a tool to offload physical and emotional frustration. You may find this exercise very releasing.

1. Lie back on your bed or sofa or some other soft surface for this exercise.

2. Pretend you are a spoiled child and simply throw a huge tantrum.

3. Continue the exercise until you either feel better or become tired or until it no longer feels comfortable.

4. Rest for a few moments then note your experiences.

The Noise-Loosening Exercise

This exercise is effective for releasing tension in your vocal cords, especially for those who use their voice professionally, or those who have throat problems. The exercise is also great for those who have difficulty finding their own voice at times. As with most offloading exercises, some degree of privacy is required.

1. You simply make infant or baby noises as they come to you organically. Resist the temptation to self-edit. For instance, if you feel you were prevented from doing something as a small child, do it now.

2. Continue until you feel better or tire. Note you experiences.

The Motor-Loosening Exercise

This intentional or offloading exercise is great for offloading muscle tension. Some people experience this tension as an urge to move during AT exercises.

Some find this offloading exercise useful before AT practice. HOWEVER THIS <u>MUST</u> ALWAYS BE DONE AT LEAST ONE (1) HOUR BEFORE ANY STANDARD AT PRACTICE SESSION. It has been found to be helpful for those who may have difficulty maintaining concentration after AT exercises.

1. Stand up and close your eyes.

2. Do a quick upward SCAN ONLY [while mentally noting any especially tense area(s)].

3. Open your eyes.

4. Gently move and shake all the areas of your body, but focusing on those areas that are especially tense for a few moments until you feel tension released from your body in general and the specific area in particular.

5. If you notice that tension remains, continue the exercise, if comfortable. If you feel better, move forward with your day or complete an AT session when appropriate.

ANXIETY & FEAR OFFLOADING EXERCISE

When we are frightened, anxious, scared, or simply need to offload worries or anxieties from the past, this exercise is effective. One of the great things about offloading exercises is that you often emerge feeling fresher, newer, and more full of optimism.

Prior to beginning the exercise, it is useful to create or retrieve a list of people, places, or situations that create anxiety-filled situations or images for you. Also, it is a good idea to limit your contact with each source of fear or anxiety until you develop the tools to deal with them in a healthier manner if possible.

1. Begin by sitting in a non-AT position as you think of people, events, or situations from your list.

2. Then, loudly verbalize any thoughts or feelings that come up for you (if you can specifically identify the source, call it by name). Whatever phrase comes up for you, simply repeat it over and over again until you eventually are quietly mumbling the phrase.

3. The point of the exercise is to expose what has been a largely unconscious event to the light of conscious awareness.

4. Continue to work through your list of fears and anxieties.

FORGIVENESS OFFLOADING EXERCISE

For many, one of the most difficult things to do is to forgive others who we believe have caused us pain or caused us loss. Invariably, all of us have suffered either physically, emotionally, or psychologically at the hands of others (or at least we believe we have). Ironically, most of us need to forgive ourselves above all.

The great lesson here is that we can only find a true peace of mind when we free ourselves from these negative emotions. When we are able to release ourselves from these ugly memories of pain, resentment, and recrimination, our lives take on a new tenor, a lightness, and a newness.

Through the process of AT, we find ourselves more open than perhaps ever before to the possibility of forgiveness. As we begin to embrace the fact that we have the choice to let go of the past, we also realize and understand we can free ourselves from this self-imposed prison as we move toward freedom from bitterness, guilt, anger, and resentment. For me and for countless others, at one moment you realize you no longer need to hang onto these negative and painful emotional past experiences. It is at this moment that you will be able to truly forgive and you will then break free of the chains of the past.

For this exercise, some find it helpful to have their favorite baseball cap, teddy bear, or whatever has been the sole witness and comforter at their moments of greatest need or vulnerability.

1. Get into a comfortable non-AT position either lying or sitting.

2. Hold or imagine holding your favorite object in your arms as you begin to rock gently back and forth.

3. You then simply say all the comforting and forgiving thoughts that come into your mind. Allow the words to simply come up.

4. Continue until you feel empty of all that needs to be said.

5. If you are able, close this chapter of your life experience. If not, continue to forgive until you are prepared to let go. If you need help, professional or otherwise, seek it out.

SADNESS OFFLOADING EXERCISES

When was the last time you experienced a really great cry? Tears, as I mentioned earlier, have a place in all of our lives. They exist to assist us in ridding ourselves of grief and sadness. Earlier, I touched on how we too often exist within constricted social norms and narrowly defined gender roles as human beings. This creates a huge gap between our free expression of a full range of emotions and the reality of our everyday lives. In other words, there is often every reason why we should cry, but we don't. This is the case even in the face of intense emotional and psychological distress.

This all-too-oft repressed need to cry plays itself out in very real symptoms. For example, in the form of incessant depression, low-energy, and early waking. There are also symptoms that are not usually associated with sadness. For instance, neck ache, joint inflammation, backache, frontal headaches, and rheumatoid arthritis. In women, it is believed that this area of unresolved emotional material may be somehow related to heavier blood loss.

Emotions may be amongst our most complex aspect as humans. Virtually nothing is cut and dried when it comes to our emotional lives. As Dr. Candice Pert says, "We are our emotions." Furthermore, emotions are often interlinked and the offloading categories used in this book only serve as broad placeholders to describe a complex landscape of endless emotional possibilities. Consider depression. It may be due, in part, to repressed rage and anger versus sadness. This underscores the further necessity of experiencing all of these offloading exercises.

Perhaps the most valuable point I can make here is for you to give yourself permission to fully experience emotions whether anger or sadness or feeling down or miserable. At the same point in time, it is just as important to then make a decision to take some action toward letting go of the associated feelings.

111

I also want to note that for all of you that "don't cry" - this exercise does not require that you actually shed an actual tear (it is more effective, but not required). This is referred to as "dry crying," which results in a very similar emotional release as the 'real' thing. Again, my perspective on this is that crying is a natural and healthy process, a gift that we should avail ourselves of often.

There are four (4) CRYING RULES that MUST BE ALWAYS OBSERVED:

1. NEVER PRACTICE the crying exercise within one (1) hour before an AT exercise. Afterwards is perfectly fine, but remember to cancel the AT session first. The reason it is not advised to do the crying exercise before an AT session has to do with not wanting to bring those feelings into an AT session.

2. NEVER PRACTICE A CRYING EXERCISE IN AN AT POSITION.

3. NEVER PRACTICE A CRYING EXERCISE BEFORE GOING TO BED.

4. NEVER PRACTICE A CRYING EXERCISE WHEN SHORT ON TIME.

The Moaning Exercise

For those who may have any difficulty with the notion of crying, this may be a useful exercise as an alternative. The exercise, as you might imagine, involves a lot of moaning, groaning, and other sounds of distress. Additionally, it is an effective tool for addressing both depression and sadness, it has also been useful for pain relief.

1. First, sit forward in your chair with your hands resting on your thighs and your eyes closed.

2. Then, gently begin to rock back and forth.

3. Begin to hum, moan, groan, or make any sound of distress that comes to mind. Continue this either until you feel empty of any sadness or until you begin to actually cry.

The Crying Exercise

Only you know and recognize when and how much you need to cry. I have talked much about the value of crying both emotionally and physically. It is a gift to yourself, treat is as such.

1. Sit comfortably on the front of your seat. For many, the best seat is the most private one in a private secure bath or while in the shower.

2. Then, pretend that you are an actor on stage having just heard some horrible news. The objective here is to cry uncontrollably using the muscles of your face, neck, shoulders, upper arms, and chest. When we have had a "really good" cry, we feel as though we have had a great workout because of the numbers of muscles we utilize in the process.

3. Repeat this a couple of times if possible.

THE BREATHING EXERCISE

Not unlike the heartbeat exercise, this breathing exercise may present special challenges to those with respiratory disease and conditions such as bronchitis, emphysema, and asthma. Those who have experienced a near-death incident involving breathing trauma such as, near-drowning, choking, or attempted strangulation may also need to proceed with extra care. Just as with the heartbeat exercise, these persons may want to introduce the formula once and to make a determination about going forward from there. Gauge your response and adjust the number of repetitions from that point.

Before we move into this week's breathing exercise, there are a few comments I would like to offer regarding the previous exercise, the heartbeat. If you did experience difficulty, then I would like to present you with the following options at this point:

1. You may proceed forward while excluding the heartbeat phrase of the formula, or

2. You may reincorporate the phrase at a later time, which will not reduce the effectiveness of the program for you. And, I want to again stress the importance of continuing to practice the offloading exercises.

Breathing itself is partly an autonomic (automatic) function and in part a fairly intentional one. As part of the AT process, muscular, vascular, and heart relaxation become integrated into the rhythm of breathing. Just as the sensations of heaviness and warmth automatically generalize from the dominant arm to other limbs, so too does breathing become a rhythmic extension within the AT process itself.

Nonetheless, *intentional modification of breathing is not desirable* as this would result in the establishment of a reflex-type mechanism. This requires being "passive" in your approach here as with all of the six standard AT exercises. In other words, you are not attempting to make or impose any voluntary change in your breathing whatsoever. This is again one of the features that distinguishes AT from yoga, where there is some breathing intentionality involved.

The exercise is being done correctly when you notice a shift from thoracic (chest) to abdominal (stomach) breathing. You can be fairly sure you are performing this portion of the exercise correctly if you breathe from your stomach. In other words, when you observe your belly rising with each breath versus your chest. Some have described a feeling similar to being lifted and lowered by an ocean wave.

Most people are familiar with any number of meditative or relaxation techniques that involve breathing as an integral part of the relaxation process. In many of these, conscious alteration in breathing patterns is used, sometimes extensively. However, breathing is utilized in a totally different manner in AT. Here, you are *not attempting to do anything* but passively observe what is going on.

The breathing formula phrase itself is indicative of this approach. It is, "It breathes me." As has been the pattern, this phrase will be inserted between the 'heartbeat' and 'neck and shoulders formulas'. It is further useful to note that since you will not be doing anything with your breathing, your objective is to:

. just focus on the rising and falling of your abdominal area,

, sub-vocally going through the formula, and

. to be mindful of the breath exiting your nostrils or mouth while continuing to passively observe what is going on in your mind/ body.

PROVIDED THAT YOU ARE HAVING NO DIFFICULTY AT THIS POINT IN YOUR AT, you may begin to proceed WITHOUT CANCELING BETWEEN SETS. The purpose of this change is to begin to allow you to go deeper in your relaxation. You may gradually increase the time and depth of your sessions at your own discretion now. At this point, you may be at the point where you are able to practice in public spaces such as parks, transit systems, your personal office, or waiting rooms.

Additionally, you may remain in any part of the formula (i.e., the heartbeat or the neck and shoulders) as you desire. You are able to prolong this time in a couple of ways:

1. By simply repeating the phrase for as long as you desire before completing the exercise, or

2. When you are in a deeply relaxed state of mental silence, you may remain there until your mind begins to wander, when this happens simply complete the exercise as usual. This is acceptable and is representative of passive concentration versus forms of regimented programming.

Finally, from this point onward, as you go deeper into relaxation, you may get in touch with colors or lights in your mind's eye. These may be experienced as exploding fireworks or colored shapes or patterns. This may expand throughout your entire field of vision or you are likely to have a completely unique experience. If this should occur, you may continue without canceling, as this only means that you have reached a deeper state of relaxation. As usual, cancel immediately if you see moving concrete images.

EXERCISE SIX

BREATHING FORMULA

1. AT position

2. Scan

3. Take your mind to your dominant arm and repeat the following:

"MY RIGHT (LEFT) ARM IS HEAVY."

"MY ARMS & LEGS ARE HEAVY & WARM." X 3

"MY HEARTBEAT IS CALM & REGULAR." X 3

"IT BREATHES ME." X 3

"MY NECK & SHOULDERS ARE HEAVY." X 3

"I AM AT PEACE." X 3

4. Note your experiences in your notebook. Repeat the exercise at your own discretion. Practice three (3) times during the day.

5. Cancel. **BUT, DO NOT CANCEL THE NIGHTLY SESSION JUST BEFORE GOING TO SLEEP AT THIS POINT IN YOUR AT.**

ABDOMINAL WARMTH

This exercise, abdominal warmth, will focus on the solar plexus region. In fact, at this point in your training you have been indirectly accessing it through the heartbeat exercises. The solar plexus is the center of the autonomic nervous system. Some believe that through focusing on this area many of the positive effects of AT (i.e., self-regulation and self-healing) are produced.

This area represents the deepest level at which you can store emotional material. Because of its importance, it is useful to describe its location and function in more detail. The solar plexus is located approximately at the top of your abdomen - in the lower chest area. It covers quite a large area and is unfamiliar to most.

If you place a finger on the soft area at the top of your abdomen, at the point where the two halves of your rib-cage meet, then mentally draw a straight line between there and an equivalent point on your back, the mid-point back is approximately where the solar plexus is located. If you happen to be a small adult, this will be about 4 inches from front to back. It surrounds both the esophagus and the aorta. Moving outward from it are nerves that extend to all vital organs of the body. These nerves involve the function of your heart, stomach, bowels, lungs, bones, muscles, arteries and veins.

The solar plexus can be thought of as the headquarters of your autonomic nervous system, which is the control panel for all the information being exchanged between the brain, organs, and tissues via the vagus nerve. It is along this complex pathway that hormones are released, organs are controlled, and the immune system is mediated. Being able to get in touch with this area allows one to indirectly affect brain function and by extension, everything else in the body.

It is important to note the appropriate precaution with respect to any stomach problems you may be experiencing at present or have experienced in the past. As always, you should consult you physician regarding this matter. Assuming no organic origin exists, Autogenic theory considers that this area stores significant emotional memories and material.

If you experience strong stomach reactions, then you can either reduce the number of repetitions or change the formula from, "My solar plexus is warm," to "My solar plexus is slightly warm."

Finally, independent of your individual experience with AT thus far, you may begin having vivid dreams and/or nightmares as your unconscious continues to offload. Of course, if these become too intense and uncomfortable, you can make the following changes.

Try using the phrase only once before gradually increasing the number of repetitions as your comfort level increases. Or, you may simply leave that section of the formula out for a short time or permanently. Again, this will not affect your overall outcome. The likely impact of this decision is to prolong the length of the process. But as you are aware at this juncture, this is not a sprint.

The abdominal warmth formula is primarily focused on relaxation of the organs. Imagery that may be helpful to you is that of a sun with its rays extending outwardly into the far reaches of the body with each exhalation. Because the solar plexus is the deepest level believed to store emotional material, you may initially experience the area as cold and/or as black. It may even feel hollow. Some people experience it as a tight ball or knot. This may be especially true if you carry much of your emotional material or memories in this area.

The key here is to be patient and stay with the process. Eventually, you will begin to feel warmth in the area. I did and you will also as countless others have. "How long," you ask? I don't know, but some have taken up to several months. All of us have our own luggage, some more, some less, but we all have unfinished business to address.

EXERCISE SEVEN

ABDOMINAL WARMTH

1. AT position

2. Scan

3. Focus your attention on your dominant arm while you become a passive observer of what happens as you go through the following formula:

"MY RIGHT (LEFT) ARM IS HEAVY."

"MY ARMS & LEGS ARE HEAVY & WARM." X 3

"MY HEARTBEAT IS CALM & REGULAR." X 3

"IT BREATHES ME." X 3

"MY SOLAR PLEXUS IS WARM." X 3

"MY NECK & SHOULDERS ARE HEAVY." X 3

"I AM AT PEACE." X 3

4. Repeat the exercise at your own discretion at this point. Note your experiences briefly.

NOTE: At this point in your training, you do not have to follow the formula by repeating three of each phrase. Follow your own sense at this juncture. Trust yourself. What you may find is yourself drifting automatically from one phrase into the next. For instance, you simply become aware of your breathing or of your heartbeat *just before the upcoming phrase in the formula.*

EXERCISE EIGHT

COOL FOREHEAD

Before beginning this exercise here are some potential challenges you may face. On occasion, some clients have reported experiencing sleep difficulties. Also, there have been reports of dizziness, which are usually short-lived and tend to disappear immediately after canceling.

IT IS VERY IMPORTANT TO UNDERSTAND THAT YOU NEVER WANT TO APPROXIMATE ANYTHING APPROACHING "COLD" WITH THIS FORMULA as it may result in a severe headache. Independent of whether or not you achieve the cool forehead experience, it is still possible to end up experiencing a headache. From an AT perspective, this may be an indication of getting in touch with emotional material, mostly sadness, which needs to be offloaded. As always, if you experience prolonged and/or unusual headaches, you should immediately consult your physician.

Furthermore, as with any standard AT exercise, you will never attempt to 'make anything happen' during the exercise. This especially applies in this cool forehead exercise. The forehead is defined as the area from one temple over to the other, above the ears and across the upper face.

If you found that during the last exercise, abdominal warmth, you either: 1) were not been able to locate your solar plexus or 2) were not able to feel any warmth in that area, you should consider spending a few more days on the abdominal warmth exercise.

However, if you determine that you should proceed forward at this time, there are a few things to consider. First, if you suffer sinus problems or catarrh, and you become aware of unbearable discomfort during practicing the exercise, you may: 1) leave the formula out while continuing to work on offloading or 2) reduce the strength of the formula by reducing the number of repetitions, or 3) adjust the wording of the formula.....

"MY FOREHEAD IS LIGHT & COOL." X 3

"MY FOREHEAD IS COOL & CLEAR." X 3

This exercise, the cool forehead, is perhaps the most difficult to achieve for the largest number of individuals who learn AT. Just as vaso-dilation results in the experience of warmth, likewise the experience of very localized vasoconstriction, reducing the blood supply, is correlated with a cooling effect.

Because the experience of a cool forehead can be quite difficult to achieve, there may be a few things that will help you in the exercise. Some find it helpful to place a cool cloth on their forehead just before the start of the exercise (removing it prior to beginning the exercise). Also, some people find it helpful to blow on the back of their hand to approximate the feeling of a cool forehead. Very few of us have access to an air-tight training room; as a result, virtually all of us will experience a slight movement of air. Even a minimal movement of air is often experienced as a cooling sensation or breeze.

EXERCISE EIGHT

COOL FOREHEAD

1. AT position

2. Scan

3. Take your attention to your dominant arm, then passively observe your body and notice what happens as you go through the following formula:

"My RIGHT (LEFT) ARM IS HEAVY."

"MY ARMS & LEGS ARE HEAVY & WARM ." X3

"MY HEARTBEAT IS CALM & REGULAR." X3

"IT BREATHES ME." X 3

"MY SOLAR PLEXUS IS WARM." X 3

"MY FOREHEAD IS COOL." X 3

"MY NECK & SHOULDERS ARE HEAVY." X 3

"I AM AT PEACE." X 3

4. Repeat the above formula (excluding the scan) as many times as you wish. The 3x3 format no longer applies to you as you may follow your own discretion.

5. Cancel (except prior to going to sleep for the evening).

Note your experiences in you notebook.

EXERCISE NINE

POSITIVE SUGGESTIONS

Congratulations! You have made it through the standard AT exercises. You have provided yourself with a magnificent gift that will provide generous returns throughout you life.

It is at this point in the practice of AT that you are able to use this deep level of relaxation to make specific changes in your personality or to rid yourself of limiting beliefs. For this purpose, positive suggestions are incorporated into the formula at this point. These are short, succinct suggestions you offer to yourself. Suggestions are always more effective when customized by you.

There are some guidelines that you should observe in creating them, however. They should always be:

. short

. simple

. positive

. present tense ("I know I am versus, I will.....")

. definitive

. by adding "I know" before any "I am" - this reinforces it.

Suggestions are goals you communicate to your unconscious. Therefore, you should focus your efforts on one suggestion at a time. By incorporating the positive suggestion into your AT practice over a period of four weeks, you can begin to determine the effectiveness of the suggestion. Based upon your results, you may wish to alter the suggestion as appropriate.

At the point where you become comfortable and have enjoyed some degree of success with a single positive suggestion, you may begin to string-together as many as three interrelated suggestions. Certain objectives such as losing weight or obesity require a multi-layered approach. For instance, you must be specific and must focus on the source of the issue to resolve it.

For example, once you have identified the source of overeating, then you are in a much better position to resolve it. Do you eat fatty and / or sugary foods because you are angry, depressed, or enraged? This is likely to require a high level of introspection, but, at this point, you will be able to access the needed internal resources to uncover the answer.

EXERCISE NINE

POSITIVE SUGGESTIONS

1. AT position

2. Scan

3. Formula:

"MY RIGHT (LEFT) ARM IS HEAVY."

"MY ARMS & LEGS ARE HEAVY & WARM." X 3

"MY HEARTBEAT IS CALM & REGULAR." X 3

"IT BREATHES ME." X 3

"MY SOLAR PLEXUS IS WARM." X 3

"MY FOREHEAD IS COOL." X 3

"I KNOW I AM_____" [repeat several times]

"MY NECK & SHOULDERS ARE HEAVY." X 3

"I AM AT PEACE." X 3

(repeat 2 - 4 times at your discretion)

CANCEL.

This approach provides a long-term benefit of the positive suggestion. You can intersperse the positive suggestion between each of the standard formulas to maximize the short-term effect of the suggestion.

Here are a few suggestions that you may find helpful. You should also be aware that suggestions will sometimes lose their effectiveness in the short term, which may necessitate changing suggestions as appropriate. Consider the following sample weight loss suggestions:

"Small frequent meals are perfect for me."

"It is easy to follow my code."

"My program is fun and simple to follow."

"I know I can stick to my program."

"I will eat my portions only."

CONCLUSION

It is my hope that you have come to realize that this is unlike the vast majority of "diet" books. I have provided you with a practical, effective approach to weight loss that is safe, simple, and sustainable. But more than that, it was my intent to help you place the 'weight' into the larger context of your life.

It is through doing so, that we are able to see it for what it is. I want to wish you the best of everything in your pursuits and in your passions from this day forward. As this is a journey, please send me digital photos and a letter to inspire others who may not yet see a clear way.

There will be someone, somewhere who will read your story or hear about it, who will see hope in your eyes, and that moment will change their lives forever. Share that gift with them as someone shared a brief moment of inspiration with you.

Nanga def, which is a west African Wolof greeting which means, "Do you have peace?" What a wonderful way for us to greet and to depart from each other.

Nanga def,

Michael Imani

Please forward all correspondence to the following address:

Dr. Michael Imani
P.O. Box 56147
Atlanta, Georgia 30343
attn: The Diet Code